# Neuroradiology Companion

## Methods, Guidelines, and Imaging Fundamentals

### Second Edition

# Neuroradiology Companion

## *Methods, Guidelines, and Imaging Fundamentals*

### Second Edition

**MAURICIO CASTILLO, M.D.**
*Professor of Radiology*
*Chief of Neuroradiology*
*The University of North Carolina School of Medicine*
*Chapel Hill, North Carolina*

LIPPINCOTT WILLIAMS & WILKINS
A **Wolters Kluwer** Company

Philadelphia • Baltimore • New York • London
Buenos Aires • Hong Kong • Sydney • Tokyo

Acquisitions Editor: Joyce-Rachel John
Developmental Editor: Brian Brown
Manufacturing Manager: Tim Reynolds
Production Manager: Kathleen Bubbeo
Production Editor: Mary Ann McLaughlin
Cover Designer: Patricia Gast
Indexer: Dorothy Jahoda
Compositor: Lippincott–Raven Desktop Division
Printer: Maple Vail

Printed in the United States of America

9   8   7   6   5   4   3   2

**Library of Congress Cataloging-in-Publication Data**

Castillo, Mauricio.
    Neuroradiology companion : methods, guidelines, and imaging fundamentals / Mauricio Castillo.—2nd ed.
        p.      cm.
    Includes bibliographical references and index.
    ISBN 0-7817-1695-0 (soft)
    1. Nervous system—Radiography—Handbooks, manuals, etc.
I. Title.
    [DNLM: 1. Central Nervous System Diseases—radiography handbooks.   2. Neuroradiography—methods handbooks.      WL 39C352n 1998]
    RC349.R3C37    1998
    616.8'04754—dc21
    DNLM/DLC
    for Library of Congress                                                  98-26851
                                                                                  CIP

*Merrick, this one is for you!*

# Contents

# Preface

*Neuroradiology Companion, Second Edition* was primarily written to help the trainee during his/her neuroradiology rotation and thus distills the most basic (and, in many respects, the most important) material in the field. The first section, "Imaging Protocols and Guidelines," contains information that trainees need to have at the ready, including basic imaging protocols, indications for invasive studies, and guidelines for contrast studies and drug usage. The second section, "Imaging Fundamentals," contains pithy, bulleted facts on the major pathological entities that one expects to encounter in daily work. These facts summarize salient clinical aspects of each of the entities, as well as key radiologic facts. The text in this section is followed by illustrations portraying the most typical imaging features of the entity as viewed through the modalities most commonly employed. Each entity is concluded with a short suggested reading list for more in-depth discovery. Every major category of CNS pathology is covered, including tumors, trauma, cerebrovascular disease and stroke, aneurysms and vascular malformations, inflammatory disease, metabolic and toxic abnormalities, congenital lesions, degenerative disc disease, and head and neck pathology. No trainee with access to this book should be stumped by a simple question. Likewise, a quick, general comparison can be made between any case in question and the image from this book; the book has functioned well as a field guide for many readers.

Some readers of the first edition offered suggestions for this one, many of which I have incorporated. All imaging protocols have been updated to reflect what I believe is state-of-the-art neuroimaging. A fairly extensive section on sedation and postsedation procedures has been added, based on those used at my institution. The treatment of adverse reactions to contrast media has been expanded and the section on what study to order has been revised in light of advances in the field. A chapter on degenerative brain disorders has been added. The text has been revised throughout, though I have made a special effort to keep the text to only the bare essentials to preserve its utility as a speedy source of information (one of the most popular features of the book). Over 95% of the illustrations are new to this edition. Most of the suggested readings have been updated, and I have tried to retain an emphasis on using readings from widely available journals and books.

*Mauricio Castillo, M.D.*

# Acknowledgments

Special thanks go to Joyce-Rachel John and James Ryan at Lippincott–Raven Publishers for their continued support of this and other projects. My daily work is facilitated by my administrative assistant, Ms. Jill Poe. My colleagues and fellows here at the University of North Carolina deserve credit for collecting many of the cases used in this book, and for allowing me the time to complete it. Thanks to Dr. Joseph Lee, Chairman of the Department of Radiology, for his continued support of the neuroradiology section.

# Part I
# *IMAGING PROTOCOLS AND GUIDELINES*

Protocols for computed tomography (CT), myelography, angiography, and magnetic resonance imaging (MRI) are provided in this section. The protocols presented may vary at different hospitals and are intended only as a guideline to help those with less experience in neuroimaging. Please use them with caution and adapt them to your particular hospital and patient needs. When in doubt, the neuroradiology trainee should always consult with the attending physician.

# 1 Computed Tomography (CT)

In *conventional* CT scanning, the collimator usually allows sections of 0.5, 1, 1.5, 3, 5, or 10 mm thickness (or more). These can be obtained contiguously, overlapping, or with an interslice gap, for example:

5-mm slices at 5-mm intervals (contiguous),
5-mm slices at 3-mm intervals (overlapping), or
5-mm slices at 10-mm intervals (gapped)

The first numeral refers to the thickness of the CT sections and the second numeral to the distance that the CT table travels after each image has been obtained. For example, when writing a protocol, one asks the technologist to perform the study at 5 × 3 mm slices. This means the slice thickness will be 5 mm with 3-mm table increments. Therefore the slices overlap each other by 2 mm. This convention applies only to conventional CT scanning.

We now use spiral (helical) CT for most studies of the brain, spine, and neck. In spiral CT scanning, the collimator allows acquisition of sections 2 to 10 mm thick, and the table moves a similar distance per second. The *pitch* refers to the relation between the slice thickness and the table increments. For example, at a pitch of 1, the table travels in 1 second a distance equal to the selected slice thickness (i.e., in 30 seconds at a slice thickness of 5 mm, a distance 150 mm in length is covered). Some spiral CT scanners allow for a pitch greater than 1; for example, at a pitch of 2, the table travels twice the distance of the slice thickness (i.e., in 30 seconds at a slice thickness of 5 mm, an area 300 mm in length is covered). Remember that as the pitch increases, the signal-to-noise ratio decreases, producing "noisier" images. Most CT units allow for total scanning times usually between 30 and 45 seconds, or back-to-back volume acquisition.

The contrast medium used for neuro CT is generally 60% iodinated material. Either ionic or nonionic contrast medium may be used, depending on the individual clinical practice. Contrast medium (total of 100 ml) for head studies is delivered with a power injector. For scanning of the neck, 150 ml of 60% iodinated contrast medium is given through power injector. For all spiral CT studies, contrast medium is given at a rate as close to 2 ml per second as possible. At my institution, we begin acquisition of all spiral CT studies 20 seconds after the beginning of the infusion of contrast medium.

## Brain

CT scans of the head generally are obtained 10 to 20 degrees from Reid's baseline (infraorbital rim to top of external auditory meatus) or parallel to the hard palate. Soft-tissue views of the posterior fossa are presented with a window width of 110 to 120 Hounsfield units (HU) and a center (level) of 43 HU. In the supratentorial region, a window width of 80 HU and a center of 43 HU are helpful. Bone windows are presented with a width of 3500 HU and a center of 700 HU. These parameters are based on the most current Siemens Somatom series of CT scanners and should be optimized for machines from other manufacturers.

1. Routine noncontrast CT scan of brain: spiral 5-mm images from base of skull to vertex.

2. Routine contrast CT scan of brain: same as for noncontrast CT scan but with the addition of 100 ml of 60% iodinated contrast material delivered at 2 ml per second as a bolus (if a precontrast study is needed, we examine the entire brain using spiral 10-mm images before administering the contrast medium).

3. Craniosynostosis: spiral CT, acquisition at 5 mm (pitch = 1), reconstruction at 3 mm, three-dimensional (3-D) reformations with conventional bone windows, then axial sections processed with high-resolution bone filter. Brain window axial views also needed.

## Spine

CT studies of the spine are presented with bone windows with a width of 4000 HU and a center of 700 HU. Soft-tissue windows are presented with a width of 400 HU and a center of 50 HU. These values are not absolute and may have to be optimized in some instances. The same values apply to spinal CT studies performed after myelography. We now perform most studies of the spine with spiral acquisition (for very large patients we still prefer conventional acquisition).

1. Routine lumbar spine: spiral 3-mm images, from the top of L-3 to mid S-1, no angle is needed. Sagittal or 3-D reformations are optional. Same technique is used after myelography. If doubt exists, conventional 1.5-mm images angled through a disk space may be performed. Contrast enhanced CT of the lumbar spine is rarely indicated (if at all).

2. Routine cervical spine: spiral 2-mm images, C-3 to T-1 (if indicated, C-1 and C-2 also may be imaged).

3. Routine thoracic spine: spiral 3-mm images through area of interest.

4. Trauma: spiral 2-mm to 3-mm images one level above and one level below injury. Subtle fractures, especially of the cervical spine, may require 1.5-mm thick slices. If level of fracture is not known, examine entire segment of spine with 3-mm images.

## Neck

Neck studies are generally presented with soft-tissue windows with a width of 250 to 270 HU and a center of 70 to 90 HU. Bone windows are presented with a width of 3500 to 4000 and a center of 700 HU. We perform all examinations of the neck with spiral acquisition.

1. Spiral CT: acquire at 5 mm (pitch = 1), reconstruct at 3 mm. The first imaging volume includes from base of skull to hyoid bone. Give contrast medium with power injector at 2 ml per second for a total of 50 ml of 60% contrast material, and wait 20 seconds before beginning acquisition. For the second imaging volume (hyoid bone to thoracic inlet), give contrast medium with power injector at 2 ml per second for a total of 100 ml of 60% contrast material; angle slices parallel to the laryngeal ventricle.

2. Conventional CT: $3 \times 3$ mm, sella to first rib, 200 ml of 60% iodinated contrast medium delivered as a bolus at 2 ml per second with power injector. Vocal cords may be examined with 3-mm or thinner slices with no gap angled parallel to laryngeal ventricle.

3. Nasopharyngeal tumors: abbreviated study from the hyoid bone to the sella with spiral 3-mm images may be performed.

4. Laryngeal cancer: an abbreviated study from the hyoid bone to the thoracic inlet with spiral 3-mm images may be performed.

## Sinuses

Coronal CT scans of the sinonasal cavities are presented with bone windows at a width of 3500 HU and a center of 700 HU and processed prospectively with a high-resolution bone filter. We now perform all studies of the paranasal sinuses with spiral acquisition.

1. Routine CT scans of sinuses: coronal (nasal bone through sphenoid sinus) spiral 3-mm images (acquire at 3 mm and reconstruct at 3 mm) with high-resolution bone windows. No contrast medium needed. Axial (hard palate through frontal sinus) spiral 3-mm images (acquire at 3 mm and reconstruct at 3 mm) with bone and soft-tissue windows are optional and generally needed in instances of noninflammatory pathologic conditions.

## Face

1. Routine CT scans of facial bones: axial (bottom of mandible through frontal sinus) spiral 3-mm images; coronal (midnose through sphenoid sinus) spiral 3-mm images (all acquired at 3 mm and reconstructed at 3 mm).

## Orbits

1. Routine CT scans of orbit: spiral 3-mm axial and coronal images (acquire at 3 mm and reconstruct at 3 mm). If the patient cannot tolerate direct coronal imaging, reformat axial acquisition in sagittal and coronal projections. Contrast enhancement may be indicated in some instances. For children, 2-mm images may be needed.

## Temporal Bones

Conventional CT still is used for evaluation of the temporal bones. Spiral CT produces images of excellent diagnostic quality when patients are not able to tolerate the longer conventional scans. We use the same technique for children and adults.

1. Axial 1-mm images 30 degrees from a line drawn tangent from the external auditory canal to the orbital roof. Start at the temporomandibular joint (TMJ) level and acquire sections up through the top of the superior semicircular canal.

2. Coronal 1-mm images (patient prone or supine): plane is parallel to angle of mandible, TMJ through back of petrous bones. Ask technologist to magnify both sides. Contrast enhancement not necessary.

# 2 Myelography

## *General Guidelines*

1. Most patients are scheduled for myelography. If there are any emergencies, discuss the case with the neuroradiology attending staff before sending for the patient.

2. Include the following possible risks and complications on the consent form and have the patient acknowledge appropriate areas: headache; bleeding; infection; seizures; nausea; vomiting; damage to nerves; paralysis; bowel, bladder, and muscle dysfunction; allergic reaction to contrast medium; and death. If the patient has a clotting disorder or low platelets (platelets need to be at least 50,000 to perform a lumbar puncture), be especially careful. Myelography on anticoagulated patients is usually avoided, if possible.

3. Check the patient's chart for allergies, as well as whether the patient is taking any of the medications listed in Chapter 5 that may either lower the seizure threshold (although not an absolute contraindication since the introduction of nonionic hypoosmolar contrast media) or increase bleeding time.

4. One of the most common problems during a myelogram is a vasovagal reaction, i.e., the patient has nausea, sweating, cold and clammy appearance, hypotension, and bradycardia. Be prepared to treat the reaction with intravenous (IV) fluids and atropine. In some instances (particularly with young men, who seem to have more vasovagal reactions), it is advisable to place an IV line before beginning the myelogram.

5. Usually inject at L2-3. Remember that most pathologic conditions are at the L4-5 or L5-S1 levels. Stay away from higher levels because that is where the conus is located (i.e., T12-L1 or L1-2). When injecting, use the "puff method" and look for the contrast medium to flow downward with the table angled slightly caudally. If there is a question about the injection being subdural, leave the needle in, do not inject any more medium, and call attending staff. A lateral cross-table radiograph will clearly show the position of the needle and of the injected contrast medium. At my institution, we always begin with a 22-gauge spinal needle. We use a standard bevel-tip needle, but a blunt-tip needle also may be used.

6. For pediatric patients, talk with attending staff first, because general anesthesia is usually used. Find out if patient has undergone magnetic resonance (MR) imaging first. (Usually the MR imaging should be done before myelography, because it almost always answers most questions.)

7. All patients undergo a computed tomographic (CT) study after myelography. Inform the CT technologist what levels need to be scanned on the basis of the findings of the conventional myelogram.

8. Ask women about possibility of pregnancy. If unsure, obtain a urine pregnancy test stat.

9. When obtaining a cervical myelogram through the lumbar route, if you see contrast medium outlining the basilar artery along the clivus or if the patient complains of headache, tilt the patient back down, because contrast medium is going up into the head and may induce seizures.

10. Suggested use of contrast myelography for adults is shown in the following table.

## Suggested Dosage of Contrast Media for Myelography in Adults

| MYELOGRAM TYPE | CONCENTRATION OF IODINATED CONTRAST MEDIUM | SUGGESTED AMOUNT |
|---|---|---|
| Lumbar | 30% | 5–15 ml |
| Cervical | 30% | 5–10 ml |
| Thoracic | 60% | 10 ml |
| Complete | 60% | 10 ml |

11. If a complete myelogram is requested, examine the thoracic area last (unless worried about a block, which usually occurs in the upper thoracic area and is encountered when running contrast medium up to the cervical area). In cases of suspected spinal cord compression inject contrast medium to rule out cord compression before removing any cerebrospinal fluid (CSF). In the presence of a compressive lesion, removal of CSF may worsen the symptoms. However, contrast medium mixed with CSF does not hinder cytologic examination of this fluid.

12. C1-2 punctures may be done to outline the superior aspect in a region of cord compression or when lumbar access is not available (e.g., for patients with severe spondylosis). With the patient in a prone position and using cross-table fluoroscopy, introduce a 22-gauge spinal needle into the posterior third of the spinal canal at the C1-2 interspace. If the needle is in the subarachnoid space, there is always CSF return. Contrast medium is injected to fill the cervical canal completely. The amount of contrast medium needed is variable, but it is safe to stop injecting it when it reaches the inferior tip of the clivus.

## *Lumbar Myelograms*

1. Scout anteroposterior (AP) and lateral lumbar views (obtained by a technologist).

2. Three spots (shallow and steep oblique and right lateral) and three spots opposite side (shallow and steep oblique and left lateral). Lateral decubitus positioning may be helpful for patients with scoliosis.

3. Cross-table lateral views (obtained by a technologist).

4. Spot lateral flexion and extension with patient standing (for those with subluxations, spondylolysis, or any other pathologic condition that affects stability).

5. Supine AP of conus (obtained last by technologist). View of conus may also be obtained with fluoroscopic spot film. This last radiograph may be skipped if the patient has undergone a prior MR imaging study that shows the position of the conus medullaris.

## Cervical Myelograms

1. Place a number of towels (or special head holder) under chin, and take scout AP, lateral, and swimmers (obtained by technologist). Neck extension should be kept to a minimum to avoid compression of the spinal cord by osteophytes or other lesions. Development or worsening of the symptoms in this position may preclude this examination. For these patients, we have performed the cervical myelography in a lateral decubitus position.
2. Prone spot cervical spine.
3. Coned spot film of occiput and foramen magnum.
4. Spots for both cervical obliques (shallow and steep obliques also may be needed).
5. Overhead horizontal beam oblique is optional.
6. Overhead cross-table lateral and swimmers views (obtained by technologist).
   a. The two most important films in cervical myelography are the prone posteroanterior (PA) spot obtained by the radiologist and the cross-table lateral obtained by the technologist.
   b. In cervical myelography, the contrast medium dissipates fairly quickly, so the films must be taken quickly. CT follows immediately.
   c. If syringomyelia is suspected, scanning 6 hours after myelography may demonstrate filling of the cavity with contrast material. This, however, rarely is needed because most of these patients are examined with MR imaging.
   d. It is critical to perform cervical myelography with lateral fluoroscopy to assure adequate placement of the needle.

## Thoracic Myelograms

1. Scout AP, lateral, and swimmers to see upper thoracic spine (obtained by technologist).
2. Usually not just a thoracic myelogram is obtained, i.e., it is part of a complete myelographic examination.
3. Injection of contrast material may be done with the patient in the lateral decubitus position with the head elevated and the shoulder braced so that contrast medium goes to the thoracic area first and not to the lumbar area, because this dilutes the contrast medium. Contrast material can be guided fluoroscopically, but may become diluted.
4. Lateral PA spots.
5. Right and left lateral decubitus cross-table, PA horizontal beam, and supine PA overhead films (obtained by technologist).
6. If block is encountered, mark the upper and lower levels of the block on the skin surface with a permanent marker to aid in radiation therapy or surgery.

7. If a complete block is encountered, a C1-2 puncture may be needed to outline the superior margin of block. However, CT usually shows some contrast medium cephalad to many "blocks."

## Postmyelography Orders

Printed orders are available in many radiology departments. If orders are handwritten, be sure to include the following:

1. Seizure precautions for 8 hours.
2. Keep head elevated at least at 45 degrees for 8 hours or until discharge, if outpatient.
3. Encourage oral (PO) fluids for 8 hours.
4. Avoid for 48 hours phenothiazines, tricyclics, monoamine oxidase (MAO) inhibitors, and other drugs that lower seizure threshold.
5. If the patient is an outpatient and the myelogram was obtained in the morning, we generally discharge the patient and let him or her go back home in the late afternoon (usually after about a 4-hour to 6-hour period of observation).

## Postmyelography Headache

1. Headache is the most common complication of myelography.
2. The headache is occipital or frontal and is postural, relieved by lying supine, exacerbated by sitting or standing, and may be accompanied by nausea, vomiting, visual disturbances, tinnitus, and hearing difficulties.
3. The headache is caused by persistent drainage of CSF through the puncture site, which results in compensatory dilatation of pain-sensitive intracranial structures.
4. Most headaches begin in the first 48 hours after the procedure and last 3 to 5 days.
5. For mild headaches, bed rest and symptomatic treatment are used.
6. For severe or persistent headaches, more aggressive symptomatic treatment and an epidural blood patch may be used. An epidural blood patch results in improvement of symptoms for more than 80% of patients. At my institution, the epidural blood patch is given by the anesthesiologists, but in other centers the radiologists administer this treatment.

**Suggested Reading**
Peterman SB. Postmyelography headache: a review. *Radiology* 1996;200:765.

# 3 Angiography

## *General Guidelines*

1. The persons performing the angiographic procedure should review the patient's chart and familiarize themselves with the patient's problems. Particular attention should be paid to prior noninvasive neurovascular studies (i.e., magnetic resonance angiography (MRA), computed tomographic angiography (CTA), and sonography).

2. Consent should be obtained before the patient is brought to the angiography suite. Risks and complications include bleeding, infection, damage to nerves and blood vessels, paralysis, difficulty with speech and vision, stroke, allergic reaction, and death.

3. If the patient is on heparin drip, have the drip discontinued approximately 4 hours before the angiogram to allow the patient's prothrombin time (PT) and partial thromboplastin time (PTT) to normalize. If possible, oral anticoagulants should be discontinued ideally 7 days (minimum 3 days) before the procedure and then the PT and PTT checked. If the angiogram is needed on an emergency basis, fresh frozen plasma has to be administered to the patient. For patients taking aspirin, bleeding time also should be obtained.

4. If previous allergic reactions have been severe (involving respiratory or cardiovascular system or angioneurotic edema), arrange for an anesthesiologist to stand by.

5. Assess patient's femoral, popliteal, and dorsalis pedis pulses, and as a rule puncture the groin with the strongest pulse. At my institution we generally puncture the right side because of the setup of the angiographic equipment. If the patient has hemiplegia, puncture the paralyzed side because it will be least prone to motion after angiography.

6. Always inject first the vessels believed to best demonstrate the pathologic condition.

7. Because of varying magnifications on digital subtraction equipment, we tape a dime to the head of the patient (any coin will serve this purpose if its diameter is known). The diameter of a dime is 18 mm.

8. As a rough rule, most neuroangiographic catheters measure 90 to 120 cm in length. Use of the following preformed catheters is suggested in the following situations:

    a. Digital arch—5 Fr (French) pigtail (however, any other 5-Fr single endhole catheter being used usually suffices).

    b. Nondigital arch—5 or 7 Fr pigtail with multiple side holes.

c. Cerebral angiogram for young adult patient—5 Fr or 7 Fr Berenstein, H1H, or JB2.

d. Cerebral angiogram for older patient—5 or 7 Fr Simmons 1, 2, or 3; H1H; or Berenstein.

e. If you cannot get a vessel before switching catheters, try a different wire first, e.g., J wire, curved wire, LLT, or glide wire.

f. When having problems with the following:

   i. Left vertebral artery, try using H1H or Berenstein catheters.

   ii. Left common carotid artery (CCA), try using a Newton or Simmons 1 or 2 catheter.

   iii. Right vertebral artery may not be possible if vessels are very tortuous. May require injection into innominate artery with distal blood pressure cuff inflated.

   iv. Glide (hydrophilic) wires and catheters are very helpful for tortuous vessels.

g. In carotid stenoses evaluation, consider a reverse-curve catheter, such as a Simmons 2 or 3, to avoid passage of guide wire to or through the stenotic bifurcation area. Be careful to avoid formation of "knots."

9. We use nonionic contrast medium for all neuroangiograms. Although conventional contrast medium may be used, nonionic contrast medium is recommended for patients with prior allergies, diabetes mellitus, heart failure, sickle cell anemia, renal insufficiency, spinal angiography, external carotid artery angiography, and interventional procedures. Suggested injection rates and sequences for cerebral angiography for children and adults are listed in the following tables.

a. Adults

## Suggested Injection Rates and Sequences for Plain-Film Cerebral Angiography for Adults

| VESSEL INJECTED | INJECTION RATE | TOTAL INJECTION |
|---|---|---|
| Arch | 20 ml/s | 60–80 ml |
| Common carotid artery | 8–10 ml/s | 10–12 ml |
| Vertebral artery | 4–6 ml/s | 6–8 ml |
| Selective internal carotid artery | 6 ml/s | 10 ml |
| Selective External carotid artery | 2–3 ml/s | 6 ml |

*Filming sequence is two to four frames per second using digital subtraction equipment. If rotational digital angiography is used, higher doses of contrast material and longer injections are needed. Vascular malformations and other high-flow lesions may require faster filming rates. Severely stenotic or occluded vessels may require slower filming rates.*

   i. For digital angiography, contrast medium may be diluted by half with normal saline solution; injection rate also may be halved. However, this suggestion may have to be optimized according to the sensitivity of the equipment being used.

   ii. Flow and film rates may need adjustment, depending on the degree of stenosis and size of vessels.

b.  Children

## Suggested Injection Rates and Sequences for Plain-Film Cerebral Angiography for Children

| | PATIENT'S WEIGHT | | | |
|---|---|---|---|---|
| VESSEL INJECTED | *>10 kg* | *10–20 kg* | *20–40 kg* | *>40 kg* |
| Internal carotid artery | 2–3 ml | 4–6 ml | 6–7 ml | 8 ml |
| External carotid artery | 1 ml | 2–3 ml | 3–4 ml | 7–8 ml |
| Common carotid artery | 4–5 ml | 5–7 ml | 6–8 ml | 9–10 ml |
| Vertebral artery | 1–3 ml | 3–4 ml | 4–5 ml | 5–6 ml |

  i.  Dosage may have to be tailored; remember children have a very dynamic flow and may require slightly higher doses than adults.
  ii.  Amounts of contrast medium in the table are the *total* dosage and have to be given over 2 to 3 seconds.
  iii.  Filming rates may have to be faster than for adults.
  iv.  If the patient is intubated, hyperventilation may slow cerebral blood flow and result in higher-quality films.

10. Do not premedicate for cerebral angiograms, because it is difficult to monitor neurologic status if the patient is sedated. Patients who are to be sedated should be asked for informed consent before a procedure.

11. If a patient reports stroke-like symptoms, do not perform further catheter manipulations. Pull the catheter out of the vessel to a position in the lower descending aorta, call neuroradiology attending staff, and call the clinician treating the patient. We generally transport these patients to the magnetic resonance (MR) imaging unit and perform diffusion-weighted imaging to rule out an infarction.

12. Make sure all patients undergo the following laboratory tests before cerebral angiography (in healthy appearing patients younger than 55 years of age, these tests may not be needed):
   a.  BUN, serum creatinine (normal: 8 to 20 mg/dL, 0.8 to 1.0 mg/dL)
   b.  PT, PTT (normal: 10 to 12.4 seconds, 21.5 to 31.9 seconds)
   c.  Bleeding time (total clotting time; normal: 9.8 to 14.0 seconds)
   d.  Hb, HCT, and platelets (normal: 13.4 to 17.4 g/dL, 40% to 54%, and 150 to 440).

13. In *preangiogram note,* briefly describe the following:
   a.  The reason for angiogram and what the computed tomographic (CT) scan, MR angiogram, or carotid Doppler sonogram showed (if the patient has undergone these studies).
   b.  Significant medical history (e.g., diabetes, hypertension, or migraine).
   c.  Allergies.
   d.  Laboratory values listed in 12. (If not already available, order the necessary tests.)

    e.  Status of patient's peripheral pulses and whether there are any carotid bruits (if you have a stethoscope handy).

    f.  Report whether the procedure was explained to the patient with the risks and benefits, including, but not limited to, bleeding, infection, damage to the nerves and vessels, paralysis, difficulty with speech and vision (i.e., stroke) and death. Indicate whether the patient's questions were answered and whether he or she gave oral and written consent (signed, witnessed, and placed in the chart).

    g.  If the patient is not capable of giving consent for the angiogram (e.g., is comatose) and no immediate family is available, consult primary or referring physician and hospital policies for such emergencies.

    h.  Have consent form witnessed.

14. If patient has hypertension, the diastolic blood pressure must be less than 110 mm Hg (if above, a cerebral angiogram is contraindicated because it will be difficult to stop bleeding from the puncture site after the catheter is removed).

15. For young women, check for the possibility of pregnancy. If unsure, perform a pregnancy test immediately.

16. Many radiology departments have printed preangiogram orders. The following are suggested if these are not available:

    a.  Only clear liquids after midnight, nothing by mouth (NPO) 2 hours before procedure.

    b.  Void before being called to radiology department.

    c.  Shave and prepare site of expected puncture (this is sometimes done in the radiology department).

    d.  Start intravenous (IV) fluids before angiogram, 1/2 normal saline solution at 75 mL/hour.

    e.  If not already available, order BUN and creatinine clearance, PT and PTT, bleeding time, Hb and HCT, and platelet tests.

17. For vasculitis evaluation, start by injecting one internal carotid artery (ICA). If this artery is abnormal, the study may be stopped, if the ICA is normal, continue with other vessels.

18. For carotid stenosis, image right anterior oblique arch, a minimum of frontal and lateral views of the neck, and frontal and lateral views of the head (to evaluate the ICA siphon).

19. For aneurysm evaluations:

    a.  May need to perform cross-compression of the ICA opposite the one being injected (if there is no cross-over flow through the anterior communicating artery to opposite anterior cerebral artery) to better visualize the anterior communicating artery.

    b.  To better visualize the anterior communicating artery and anterior cerebral arteries near the midline, obtain an oblique view opposite to the carotid artery being injected, e.g., right ICA injection with the head turned to the left approximately 30 degrees.

20. For vertebral arteries, keep the catheter low in the vessel, and perform the test injection to observe size and flow rate. If the arteries are of medium or small size or if a decreased flow rate is found, pull the catheter out of the vessel as

soon as the injector has completed its full injection (do not wait until the film sequence is over). If the artery terminates in the posterior inferior cerebellar artery (PICA), do not inject. Manipulation of catheters in the vertebral arteries commonly results in vasospasm. In the presence of vasospasm, withdraw the catheter from that vessel. Most vasospasms resolve spontaneously in 5 to 10 minutes.

21. In the *postangiogram notes* include procedure performed, preliminary findings, complications, and status of the patient's peripheral pulses, (e.g., palpable or nonpalpable femoral, popliteal, and dorsalis pedis [DP] pulses). Also mark the DP and posterior tibialis (PT) pulses with an indelible pen on the patient's feet to help the nurses who check the vital signs and pulses after the procedure. Documentation as to the presence of an attending physician is required in the U.S.

22. Postangiogram orders may be preprinted. If not available, the following are suggested:

    a. Enforce strict bed rest with leg or arm (whichever was used) straight for 6 hours.

    b. Enforce bed rest except for bathroom needs for next 6 hours.

    c. Order normal diet, and encourage oral (PO) fluids for 12 hours.

    d. Take vital signs, and check the groin for hematoma or bleeding and pulses peripheral to puncture site every 15 minutes for 4 hours, then every 30 minutes for 4 hours, then only routine vital signs. Significant hematomas occur in 5% to 10% of all cerebral angiograms. This risk is higher in brachial and axillary punctures than in groin punctures. Hematomas judged to contain the equivalent to one unit of blood generally will require exploration of repair of the vessel.

    e. Call radiology (or neuroradiology) house officer at _____, if complications occur or with questions.

23. If patients are outpatients, we discharge them to home in the late afternoon after an observation period of 6 hours and only if they are stable.

24. The use of collagen sponge plugs may prevent the formation of a groin hematoma among patients who receive anticoagulation during angiography and is helpful for outpatients (prevents a hematoma, allowing them to be discharged as planned). We now use the Angio-Seal type of these devices. Note is made that use of these devices requires a short training period.

25. Anticoagulation during a procedure is obtained for adults by giving a bolus of 5000 units of heparin IV. The optimal activated clotting time (ACT) is 1.5 to 2.5 times that of baseline. Anticoagulation is not generally needed for diagnostic neuroangiography. Heparinization may be reversed by giving 10 mg of protamine sulfate for every 1000 units of heparin administered IV over a 10-minute period.

**Suggested Readings**

Kussmaul WG, Buchbinder M, Whitlow PL, et al. Rapid arterial hemostasis and decreased access site complications after cardiac catheterization and angioplasty: results of a randomized trial of a novel hemostatic device. *J Am Coll Cardiol* 1995;25:1685.

Morris P. *Practical neuroangiography.* Baltimore: Williams & Wilkins, 1997:1-63.

# 4 Magnetic Resonance Imaging

All the following protocols are based on a Siemens Vision 1.5T system, but they are appropriate for all modern magnetic resonance imaging (MRI) systems and are designed to be performed in less than 50 minutes. All measurements are given in milliseconds and millimeters.

## Infant Brain (Younger Than 12 Months)

| SEQ# | PLANE | TR | TE | FOV | THK/GAP | FLIP | NSA | OTHER |
|------|-------|------|--------|-----|---------|------|-----|-------|
| 1 | SAG | 600 | 15 | 220 | 4/1 | — | 1 | |
| 2 | AXIAL | 4500 | 15/105 | 200 | 4/1 | — | 1 | TSE |
| 3 | AXIAL | 600 | 15 | 200 | 4/1 | — | 2 | |
| 4 | COR | 600 | 15 | 200 | 4/1 | — | 2 | |

*Note: Try to use extremity coil for very small patients.*
*Seq, sequence; TR, repetition time; TE, echo time; FOV, field of view; Thk/Gap, slice thickness and interslice gap; Flip, flip angle; NSA, number of signal averages; TSE, turbo (fast) spin echo.*

## Noncontrast Brain for Patients Older Than 12 Months

| SEQ# | PLANE | TR | TE | FOV | THK/GAP | FLIP | NSA | OTHER |
|------|-------|------|---------|-----|---------|------|-----|-------|
| 1 | SAG | 600 | 15 | 240 | 6/1 | — | 1 | |
| 2 | AXIAL | 4000 | 15/105 | 230 | 6/1 | — | 1 | |
| 3 | COR | 4000 | 15/105 | 230 | 6/1 | — | 1 | |
| 4* | AXIAL | 0.8 | 123.0/1 | 240 | 6 | 90 | 1 | 128 × 200, B = 30 |
| 5* | AXIAL | 0.8 | 123.0/1 | 240 | 6 | 90 | 1 | 128 × 200, B = 1000–1300 |

*\*For suspected cerebral infarction, diffusion-weighted imaging (echoplanar) may be done.*
*All T2-weighted sequences obtained with turbo (fast) spin echo. B values for diffusion-weighted imaging depend on the gradients available and vary according to different manufacturers. Total acquisition time for diffusion imaging is 4 to 5 seconds.*

## Contrast Brain (Begin with Noncontrast Protocol, Then Do the Following)

| SEQ# | PLANE | TR | TE | FOV | THK/GAP | FLIP | NSA | OTHER |
|------|-------|-----|-----|-----|---------|------|-----|-------|
| 1 | AXIAL | 760 | 14 | 230 | 6/1 | — | 1* | † |
| 4 | COR | 760 | 14 | 230 | 6/1 | — | 1* | † |

*With flow compensation on, TE increases approximately 7 milliseconds and may be used except for patients with suspected strokes. This improves visualization of posterior fossa by reducing ghost artifacts from venous sinuses (in my experience, these artifacts are prominent in the Siemens unit and less prominent in units from other manufacturers). For children with posterior fossa tumors, add sagittal T1-weighted postgadolinium. Consent has to be obtained for children under 2 years of age.*
*†Magnetization transfer is used in all postgadolinium T1-weighted sequences.*

## Contrast Brain for Seizures

| SEQ# | PLANE | TR | TE | FOV | THK/GAP | FLIP | NSA | OTHER |
|------|-------|------|--------|-----|---------|------|-----|-------|
| 1 | SAG | 600 | 15 | 240 | 6/1 | — | 1 | |
| 2 | AXIAL | 4000 | 15/105 | 230 | 6/1 | — | 1 | TSE |
| 3 | COR | 4000 | 15/105 | 200 | 5/1 | — | 1* | |
| *Post GD* | | | | | | | | |
| 4- | AXIAL | 760 | 14 | 230 | 5/1 | — | — | +MT |
| 5 | COR | 760 | 14 | 230 | 5/1 | — | — | +MT |
| *For Hippocampal studies†* | | | | | | | | |
| 6 | COR | 4600 | 90 | 260 | 3/.15 | — | 2 | TSE (effective 512 × 512 matrix) |
| 7 | COR | 35 | 6 | 250 | 1.5 (total slices=124) | 35 | 1 | 192 × 256 GRE |
| 8 | COR | 9000 | 119 | 240 | 3 | 180 | 1 | 224 × 256 FLAIR, inversion time=2200 |

*†(Start at level of mammillary bodies on sagittal view, and go back as far as possible; angle perpendicular to long axis of hippocampus as seen on parasagittal images). Contrast agent is given only when a tumor in the hippocampus is suspected.*
*GD, gadolinium; +MT, with magnetization transfer; GRE, gradient echo; FLAIR, fluid-attenuated inversion recovery.*

## Sella/Pituitary Gland

| SEQ# | PLANE | TR | TE | FOV | THK/GAP | FLIP | NSA | OTHER |
|------|-------|-----|------|-----|---------|------|-----|-------|
| 1 | SAG | (brain) 600 | 15 | 240 | 6/1 | — | 1 | |
| 2 | AXIAL | (brain) 4000 | 15/105 | 230 | 6/1 | — | 1 | TSE |
| 3 | COR (sella) | 500 | 15 | 200 | 3/.1 | — | 4 | $192 \times 256$ |
| *Post GD* | | | | | | | | |
| 4 | COR (sella) | 500 | 15 | 200 | 3/.1 | — | 4 | $192 \times 256$ |
| 5 | SAG (sella) | 500 | 15 | 200 | 3/.1 | — | 4 | $192 \times 256$ |
| *Dynamic studies* | | | | | | | | |
| 6 | COR (sella) | 125 | 6 | 200 | 3 (total slices=5) | 80 | 1 | $128 \times 256$ |

Notes: Resolution (last column) is given for rectangular matrices. Magnify sella 1.5. For postcontrast studies, one-half dose gadolinium may be used with good clinical results. For dynamic studies, the measurements are repeated five times every 30 seconds.

## Internal Auditory Canals/Temporal Bones

| SEQ# | PLANE | TR | TE | FOV | THK/GAP | FLIP | NSA | OTHER |
|------|-------|-----|------|-----|---------|------|-----|-------|
| 1 | SAG (brain) | 600 | 15 | 240 | 6/1 | — | 1 | |
| 2 | AXIAL (brain) | 4000 | 15/105 | 230 | 6/1 | — | 1 | TSE |
| 3 | AXIAL (IACs) | 500 | 15 | 165 | 3/0.1 | — | 3 | $224 \times 256$ |
| *Post GD* | | | | | | | | |
| 4 | AXIAL (IACs) | 500 | 15 | 165 | 3/0.1 | — | 3 | $224 \times 256$ |
| 5 | COR (IACs) | 500 | 15 | 200 | 3/0.1 | — | 3 | $224 \times 256$ |
| *Screening with 3-D CISS.** | | | | | | | | |
| 6 | AXIAL (IACs) | 12.3 | 5.9/1 | $185 \times 185$ | 0.7 | 70 | 2 | $256 \times 512$ |

*May avoid use of contrast medium.
Notes: Magnify IACs 1.5.
IAC, internal auditory canal.
CISS, constructive interference in the steady state.

## Orbits

| SEQ# | PLANE | TR | TE | FOV | THK/GAP | FLIP | NSA | OTHER |
|------|-------|-----|-----|-----|---------|------|-----|-------|
| 1 | SAG (brain) | 520 | 15 | 240 | 5/0.2 | — | 1 | |
| 2 | AXIAL (brain) | 4000 | 15/105 | 230 | 6/1 | — | 1 | Include orbits and TSE |
| 3 | AXIAL (orbits) | 500 | 15 | 160 | 3/0.1 | — | 2 | 256 × 512 |
| *Post GD* | | | | | | | | |
| 4 | AXIAL (orbits) | 600 | 15 | 160 | 4 | — | 3 | Fat saturation pulse |
| 5 | COR (orbits) | 600 | 15 | 160 | 4 | — | 3 | Fat saturation pulse |

*Note: Fat saturation pulse averages 230 to 250. On the Vision system, it is automatically selected. Because it uses part of the TR, the number slices may be slightly reduced.*

## Cervical Spine

| SEQ# | PLANE | TR | TE | FOV | THK/GAP | FLIP | NSA | OTHER |
|------|-------|-----|-----|-----|---------|------|-----|-------|
| 1 | SAG | 500 | 150 | 280 | 4/0.1 | — | 3 | |
| 2 | SAG | 3500–4000 | 19/93 | 280 | 4/0.3 | — | 1 | TSE |
| 3 | AXIAL | 650 | 20 | 200 | 4/0.5 | 25–30 | 2–4 | GRE |

*Note: Do study with dedicated surface coil.*

## Thoracic Spine

| SEQ# | PLANE | TR | TE | FOV | THK/GAP | FLIP | NSA | OTHER |
|------|-------|-----|-----|-----|---------|------|-----|-------|
| 1 | SAG | 500 | 15 | 180 | 4/0.5 | — | 3 | 256 × 256 |
| 2 | SAG | 3500 | 93 | 280 | 4/0.3 | — | 1 | TSE, 192 × 256 |
| 3 | AXIAL | 540 | 12 | 180 | 4/0.5 | 15 | 3 | TSE, 192 × 256 |
| 4 | COR | 4000 | 93 | 220 | 5/0.3 | — | 1 | TSE, 192 × 256 |

*Note: If gadolinium is needed, do the axial and sagittal T1WI immediately after contrast is given.*

## Lumbar Spine

| SEQ# | PLANE | TR | TE | FOV | THK/GAP | FLIP | NSA | OTHER |
|------|-------|------|------|------|---------|------|------|-------|
| 1 | SAG | 500 | 15 | 250 | 4/0.5 | — | 2 | $173 \times 256$ |
| 2 | SAG | 3400 | 90 | 250 | 4/0.3 | — | 2 | TSE, $190 \times 256$ |
| 3 | AXIAL | 650 | 15 | 180 | 5/0.5 | — | 1 | $256 \times 256$* |
| 4 | AXIAL (optional) | 5300 | 120 | 180 | 4/0.5 | — | 2 | TSE, $270 \times 512$ |

*Angle through L3-4, L4-5, L5-S1, or stack from L3 to S1. For contrast-enhanced studies, repeat sequences 1 and 3 immediately after administration of the contrast material.*

## Neck

| SEQ# | PLANE | TR | TE | FOV | THK/GAP | FLIP | NSA | OTHER |
|------|-------|------|------|------|---------|------|------|-------|
| 1 | AXIAL | 690 | 15 | 200 | 4/1 | — | 2 | $192 \times 256$ |
| 2 | AXIAL | 4000 | 93 | 200 | 4/1 | — | 1 | TSE |
| *Post GD* | | | | | | | | |
| 4 | AXIAL | 690 | 15 | 200 | 4/1 | — | 2 | * |
| 5 | COR | 630 | 15 | 200 | 4/1 | — | 2 | * |

*Fat suppression imaging may be helpful.*

## MR Angiograms (Time-of-Flight)

| TYPE OF STUDY | PLANE | TR | TE | FOV | SLICES | FLIP | NSA | OTHER |
|---------------|-------|------|------|------|--------|------|------|-------|
| 3-D TOF for neck or circle of Willis* | AXIAL | 35 | 6 | 200 | Volume: 64 1-mm partitions | 20 | 1 | $192 \times 256$ superior presaturation band, +MT |
| 2-D TOF for neck or slow-flowing blood | AXIAL | 40 | 9 | 230 | 54 slices, 3 mm each | 35 | 1 | $160 \times 256$ superior presaturation (traveling band), +MT |
| 2-D TOF venogram | OBLIQUE, SAG, or COR (20 degrees) | 32 | 10 | 200 | 40–55 slices, 3 mm each | 50 | 1 | $256 \times 256$ inferior presaturation band, +MT |

*Use tilted optimized nonsaturating excitations (TONE-UP=2). TOF, time of flight.*

### Suggested Readings

For additional information on protocols for imaging of the cranial nerves:

Mukherji SK, Castillo M, Daughtry LH. MR imaging protocols for evaluation of the cranial neuropathies. *Top Magn Reson Imaging* 1996;8:187.

## COMPATIBILITY OF COMMON DEVICES AND IMPLANTS AND MAGNETIC RESONANCE IMAGING

The following is a partial list of the most common devices that may move or deflect in a magnetic field.

### *Vascular Aneurysm and Hemostatic Clips*
Downs multipositional (17-7PH)
Drake 14, 16, 24, 301SS
Heifetz 17-7PH
Housepian implant
Kapp 405SS (standard, straight, and curved)
Mayfield 301SS and 304SS
McFadden 301SS
Pivot 17-17PH
Scoville EN58J
Sundt Kees 301SS
Sundt Kees multiangle 17-7PH
Vari-angle 17-7PH
Vari-angle Micro 17-7PM SS
Vari-angle Spring 17-7PM SS

Caution: A death has resulted from torsion of an Aesculap-Yasargil aneurysm clip. Although the later generation of these devices is said to be MRI compatible, caution is advised if MRI is to be performed on any patient with an intracranial aneurysm clip.

### *Carotid Clamps*
Carotid clamps are firmly lodged, and injury to patients harboring them is unlikely.

Crutchfield SS
Kindt SS
Poppen Blaylock SS
Salibi SS
Selvertone SS

### *Heart Valves*
Heart valves move in the magnet; however, their motion is less than that exerted by normal cardiac contraction, so MRI may be considered safe with all of them.

Beall
Bjork-Shiley Universal Spherical, 25 MBRC 11030, and MBC
Carpentier Edwards 2650 and porcine
Hall Kaster A7700
Hancock 1 and 2 porcine
Hancock extracorporeal R and M4365-33
Ionescu-Shiley
Lillehi Kaster 300S and 5009
Medtronic Hall and model A7700-D-16
Omnicarbon 3523T029

Omniscience 6522
Smeloff Cutter
Starr-Edwards 1260, 2320, Pre6000, and 6520
St. Jude A101 and M101

### Cardiac Pacemakers and Implantable Cardiac defibrillators
Patients with cardiac pacemakers and implantable cardiac defibrillators should not undergo imaging.

### Implantable Drug Pumps
Patients with implantable drug pumps should not undergo imaging.

### Intravascular Devices
Intravascular devices are firmly lodged 6 weeks after implantation, and injury to patients harboring them is unlikely.

Cook occluding spring embolization coil
Gianturco Bird Nest
Gianturco embolization coils
Gianturco zig-zag stent
Greenfield vena cava filter
Gunther IVC filter
Palmaz endovascular stent
New retrievable IVC filter

### Ocular Implants
Fatio eyelid spring/wire (patients with these devices may undergo imaging if the eye is protected with a patch)
Retinal Tack SS-martensitic

### Ear Implants
3M cochlear implant
Nucleus mini 22-channel cochlear implant
McGee piston stapes prosthesis platinum/stainless steel

### Bullets
Daisy and Crossman BBs
Norinco bullet, 39 mm
Geco bullet, 0.38 inch
Evansville Ordnance bullet, 0.45 inch
Norma bullet, 9 mm
All foreign bullets should be considered ferrogmagnetic

### Penile Implants
Omniphase

### Vascular Access Devices
Vascular access devices are firmly lodged, and injury to patients harboring them is unlikely, but they may cause significant artifact.

### Biopsy Needles
18-g ASAP automatic core biopsy needle
14-g, 18-g, and 20-g Biopty-Cut needle
18-g Ultra-core

### Halo Vests
AOA ambulatory halo system
EXO adjustable collar
Guilford cervical orthosis
SOMI cervical orthosis

### Vagal Nerve Stimulators
Patients harboring vagal nerve stimulators should not undergo imaging.

### Bone growth stimulators
Patients harboring bone growth stimulators should not undergo imaging.

### Other Devices
The following devices will not injure patient despite motion or deflection in an MRI unit.

Contraceptive diaphragm
Holter type shunt valve
Vascular marker O-ring washer 302SS
Swan-Ganz catheters do not move, but one device "melted" in a patient
    undergoing MRI
Dental devices and implants are generally safe but may produce considerable artifact
Pacemakers and medication infusion pumps for pain should not be placed in the magnet

Imaging of patients with metallic fragments (e.g., history of welding) should not be performed. Screening of these patients with thin-section CT or plain radiographs of the orbits is advisable.

The foregoing lists do not include all medical implants and devices. For further information, always consult with the manufacturer of an implant or device.

Other relative contraindications to MRI include the following:

Claustrophobia
Weight over 290 lb
More than 55 cm girth at widest point
Garments using "Angelica" fabric or Freostat (>1% steel)
Oxygen face masks
Jewelry
External fixators for fractures
Cataract lens implants (especially Lynnel model)

### Suggested Reading
Shellock FG. *Pocket guide to MR procedures and metallic objects: update 1996.* Philadelphia: Lippincott-Raven, 1996.

# 5  Drugs

## Medications That May Lower Seizure Threshold

Generic names are listed in the first column, trade names are listed in the second column. Asterisk indicates that drug is used especially for its antihistaminic activity.

**PHENOTHIAZINE DERIVATIVES**

| | |
|---|---|
| chlorpromazine* Hcl | Thorazine |
| fluphenazine | Prolixin |
| mechdilazine* | Tacaryl |
| mesoridazine | Serentil |
| perphenazine | Trilafon |
| prochlorperazine* | Compazine |
| promazine Hcl | Sparine |
| promethazine* | Phenergan |
| trifluoperazine | Stelazine |
| triflupromazine Hcl | Vesprin |
| trimeprazine* | Tamaril |

**MAO INHIBITORS**

| | |
|---|---|
| isocarboxazid | Marplan |
| pargyline | Eutonyl |
| phenelzine | Nardil |
| tranylcypromine | Parnate |

**TRICYCLIC ANTIDEPRESSANTS**

| | |
|---|---|
| amitriptyline | Elavil |
| amoxapine | Asendin |
| desipramine | Norpramin |
| doxepin | Adapin, Sinequan |
| imipramine | Tofranil |
| maprotiline | Ludiomil |
| nortriptyline | Pamelor |
| protriptyline | Vivactil |

trazodone            Desyrel

trimipramine         Surmontil

**CNS STIMULANTS**

amphetamines

analeptics           No Doz, Vivarin

anorexians           Tenuate

doxapram             Dopram

**ANTIDEPRESSANTS**

fluoxetine           Prozac

methylphenidate      Ritalin

**ANTIPSYCHOTICS**

haloperidol          Haldol

lithium              Eskalith

molindone            Moban

thiothixine          Navane

# Over-the-Counter Medications That Increase Bleeding Time

**COMMON MEDICATIONS THAT CONTAIN ASPIRIN OR ITS DERIVATIVES (TRADE NAMES)**

Alka Seltzer

Anacin

Arthritis Pain Formula

Ascriptin

Aspercin

Aspergum

Bufferin

Darvon

Disalcid

Diurex

Doan's Pills

Dolcin

Dolprin #3

Drinophen

Duradyne

Easprin

Ecotrin

Excedrin

Fiorinal

Gelprin

Genprin

Gensan

Goody's powders

Infantol Pink

Lartab ASA

Magan

Magnapirin

Meprobamate

Meprogesic Q

Midol

Mobidin

Mobigesic

Momentum

Neogesic

Norwich

Pepto-Bismol

Percodan

Persistin

Propoxyphene

Rexolate

Robaxisal

Roxiprin

Salcitab

Salocol

Slatin

Supac

Talwin

Tenol-Plus

TriPain

Trisalte

Tusal

Valesin

Verin

Wesprin

Zorprin

**COMMON MEDICATIONS THAT CONTAIN NONSTEROIDAL ANTIINFLAMMATORY AGENTS (TRADE NAMES)**

Advil

Anaprox

Butazolidin

Clinoril

CoAdvil

Dolobid

Dristan Sinus

Feldene

Ibuprin

Indocin

Medipren

Menodol

Midol 200

Motrin IB

Nalfon

Naprosyn

Nuprin

Pamprin IB

Pediaprofen

Rufen

Saleto-200

Tolectin

Ultrapin

Unipro

Valprin

**Suggested Reading**

Bartley GB, Warndahl RA. Surgical bleeding associated with aspirin and nonsteroidal anti-inflammatory agents. *Mayo Clin Proc* 1992;67:402-403.

# *Medications for Reactions to Contrast Media*

1. Diphenhydramine (Benadryl)

   This antihistaminic agent produces relief of minor allergic reactions but induces drowsiness and anticholinergic effects (therefore do not use if a patient has glaucoma or prostatic hypertrophy).

   Parenteral dose (IV/IM)    Child: 1.25 mg/kg.
   Adult: 25–50 mg

   Oral dose    Child: 1.25 mg/kg q4–6h
   Adult: 25–50 mg q4–6h

2. Epinephrine

   This alpha and beta receptor agonist induces vasoconstriction and increased peripheral vascular resistance, increases cardiac output, relaxes bronchi, inhibits histamine release, and relieves pulmonary edema. Do not use in cases of preexisting beta blockade.

   Dose for mild to moderate reactions

   Concentration: 1:1000

   Route: SQ/IM

   Volume:    Child: 0.1 to 0.3 mL/kg (<0.5 mL total)
   Adult: 0.3 to 0.5 mL

| Repeat: | Child: q30 minutes |
|---|---|
|  | Adult: q15 minutes |

Dose for severe reactions

| Concentration: 1:10,000 | Route: IV over 5 minutes |
|---|---|
| Volume: | Child: 1 to 3 mL |
|  | Adult: 3 to 5 mL |
| Repeat: | Child: q30 minutes |
|  | Adult: q15 minutes |

3.  Aminophylline
    Increases cyclic adenosine monophosphate (cAMP) level, leading to bronchial muscle relaxation, central nervous system (CNS) stimulation, and cardiovascular effects. May produce hypotension and seizures.

    Dose for acute bronchospasm: 5 to 6 mg/kg IV slowly

4.  Dexamethasone sodium phosphate
    This corticosteroid is easier to use in an emergency and has the fastest effect. It inhibits production of allergic mediators.

    Dose for acute reaction: 20 mg IV q2–6h PRN

5.  Atropine
    Produces anticholinergic effects, thereby inhibiting vagal tone and is useful for bradycardia accompanied by hypotension.

    Dose for acute reactions

    Child: 0.2 mg/kg IV (<0.6 mg total)

    Adult: 0.5 to 1 mg IV q5–10 minutes (<2 mg total)

6.  Diazepam (Valium)
    This γ-aminobutyric acid (GABA) agonist inhibits neuronal firing and may be used to control seizures. It may be cardiotoxic and cause respiratory depression.

    Dose in acute situation:

    Child: 0.2 to 0.5 mg/kg IV q20–30 minutes for a maximum of two doses

    Adult: 5 to 10 mg IV q20–30 minutes

7.  Other medications, such as naloxone (Narcan), lidocaine, nitroprusside, phentolamine, ranitidine, and sodium bicarbonate, are used less often to manage reactions to contrast media and require more experience. Consult with the nurse or anesthesiologist or both for correct use.

## *Suggested Management of Acute Allergic Reactions*

| | |
|---|---|
| Urticaria | If needed, diphenhydramine (Benadryl) |
| Facial or laryngeal edema | Intubation and, if needed, epinephrine |
| Bronchospasm | Oxygen and, if needed, epinephrine; if no response, aminophylline |
| Severe hypotension | IV fluids (0.9% normal saline solution), oxygen, epinephrine; if no response, atropine |

## *Endotracheal Tubes*

| Age | Tube size (mm) |
|---|---|
| 0 to 6 months | 3.0 to 3.5 |
| 6 to 12 months | 3.5 to 4.0 |
| 12 to 24 months | 4.0 to 4.5 |
| >24 months | 16 + age in years divided by 4 |
| Adults | 6.0 to 8.0 |

## *Prevention of Reactions to Contrast Media for Patients with Allergies*

Prednisone, 50 mg PO q6h for three doses starting the day before the procedure, or

Methylprednisolone, 32 mg PO 6 to 24 hours before and then repeat dose 2 hours before procedure.

Diphenhydramine (Phenergan), 50 mg PO or IV 1 hour before procedure.

We use nonionic contrast media for all patients who have had a prior allergic reaction.

### Suggested Readings

Bettmann MA, Heeren T, Greenfield A, Goudey C. Adverse events with radiographic contrast agents: results of the SCVIR contrast agent registry. *Radiology* 1997;203:611.

Lasser EC, Berry CC, Mishkin MM, Williamson B, Zheutlin N, Silverman JM. Pretreatment with corticosteroids to prevent adverse reactions to nonionic contrast media. *AJR Am J Roentgenol* 1994;162:523.

Lasser EC, Lyon SG, Berry CC. Reports on contrast media reactions: analysis of data from reports to the U.S. Food and Drug Administration. *Radiology* 1997;203:605.

# 6 Sedation

## *Preprocedural and Intraprocedural Care*

At my institution, conscious sedation is now used routinely. It is administered by either two registered nurses or anesthesia technologists under supervision of a physician. The goals of conscious sedation are to depress only minimally the level of the patient's consciousness, to maintain a patent airway, and to allow the patient to respond to commands. Generally, emergency equipment such as oxygen, suction, monitors, Ambubag, mask, and resuscitation drugs should be readily available. The patient should have an empty stomach (adults: nothing by mouth [NPO] 4 to 6 hours before sedation; children: NPO 2 hours before sedation). During sedation, continuous monitoring of vital signs and oxygen saturation (normally greater than 95%) is needed. We record vital signs and oxygen saturation every 15 minutes. The level of consciousness of a patient is continuously evaluated and recorded every 15 minutes according to a sedation scale as follows:

| | |
|---|---|
| Fully awake | 5 points |
| Arouses easily | 4 points |
| Arouses with tactile stimuli | 3 points |
| Arouses with vigorous stimuli | 2 points |
| Arouses with painful stimuli | 1 point |
| Unresponsive | 0 points |

The following is a list of the most common drugs used for conscious sedation at our institution. This list details drugs administered intravenously. All drugs should be given slowly.

### PARENTERAL DRUGS

### Pentobarbital Sodium (Nembutal)

This medication is used for sedation. It is probably the medication we use most. It causes rapid sedation given through either IV or IM routes. Its side effects include respiratory and cardiovascular depression. Use of pentobarbital sodium should be avoided in the care of patients with hepatic insufficiency. If given IV the onset of pentobarbital is immediate; when given IM the onset is within 10 to 15 minutes. The effect lasts 15 to 20 minutes. We do not use pentobarbital sodium in the care of children younger than 6 months.

| Age | Dose |
|---|---|
| Children | 2 mg/kg/dose IV (repeat dose of 1 mg/kg up to maximum of 7 mg/kg, not to exceed total of 500 mg) |

| Children | 2 to 6 mg/kg IM (maximum dose of 100 mg) |
|---|---|
| Adults | 100 mg IV (repeat in equal increments up to maximum of 500 mg) |
| Adults | 150 to 200 mg IM |

### Morphine sulfate

Morphine is used for sedation and to manage severe pain. Use may cause nausea and vomiting and respiratory depression. Its antagonist is Narcan. Morphine should not be given to patients with increased intracranial pressure or respiratory depression. The effect of morphine peaks 20 to 60 minutes after administration and may last 3 to 5 hours.

| Age | Dose |
|---|---|
| Neonates | 0.05 mg/kg IV |
| Infants and children | 0.05 to 0.1 mg/kg/dose (may be repeated up to maximum of 15 mg) |
| Adolescents | 3 to 4 mg IV (may be repeated up to maximum of 15 mg, increments of 1.2 mg) |
| Adults | 10 mg IV (may be repeated up to maximum of 20 mg, increments of 1 to 2 mg) |

### Fentanyl

Fentanyl is used to manage pain and for sedation. It may cause side effects similar to those of morphine, and its antagonist is also Narcan. The onset of fentanyl is immediate, and its effects last 30 to 60 minutes.

| Age | Dose |
|---|---|
| Infants and children | 1 to 2 µg/kg IV (may be repeated up to maximum dose of 5 µg/kg, increments of 1 µg/kg) |
| Adults | 0.5 to 1 µg/kg IV |

### Meperidine (Demerol)

Meperidine (Demerol) is used to treat patients with moderate-to-severe pain. Its side effects are similar to those of morphine and its antagonist is Narcan. The onset of action of meperidine occurs within 5 minutes of administration, and the effect lasts 2 to 4 hours.

| Age | Dose |
|---|---|
| Children | 1 to 1.5 mg/kg/dose IV (maximum initial dose of 100 mg, maximum total dose of 150 mg, increments of 1 mg/kg) |
| Adults | 50 to 150 mg/dose IV |

### Midazolam (Versed)

Midazolam (Versed) is used for sedation. It may cause cardiac and respiratory depression. Its antagonist is flumazenil. The onset of action is within 1 to 5 minutes after administration, and the effect lasts 2 to 6 hours.

| Age | Dose |
|---|---|
| Children | 0.05 mg/kg/dose IV (maximum initial dose of 2 mg, maximum total dose of 5 mg) |

| | |
|---|---|
| Adults | 0.5 to 2 mg IV (repeat every 3 minutes for maximum dose of 5 mg) |

**Diazepam (Valium)**

The indications, antagonist, and onset of action of diazepam are similar to those of midazolam. The duration of effect is 1 to 2 hours.

| Age | Dose |
|---|---|
| Children | 0.05 mg/kg/dose IV (maximum initial dose of 5 mg, maximum total dose of 10 mg) |
| Adults | 5 mg IV (may be repeated for maximum dose of 10 mg) |

**Lorazepam (Ativan)**

The indications and antagonist of lorazepam are similar to those of midazolam. The onset of action is 15 minutes, and the effect lasts 30 to 180 minutes.

| Age | Dose |
|---|---|
| Children | 0.05 mg/kg/dose IV (maximum dose of 2 mg) |
| Adults | 2 mg IV (maximum dose of 4 mg) |

ORAL DRUGS

For children younger than 2 years, we begin by giving oral sedation. If this type of sedation fails, we administer parenteral sedation. These medications should be given 30 to 60 minutes before the procedure.

**Chloral Hydrate**

This drug is used for nonpainful procedures. Its side effects include gastrointestinal upset and paradoxic excitement. Use of chloral hydrate is contraindicated in the care of patients with liver or renal insufficiency. The effect peaks 30 to 60 minutes after administration and may last up to 8 hours. The drug also may be given per rectum.

| Age | Dose |
|---|---|
| Neonates | 25 mg/kg/dose by mouth (PO) or rectally |
| Children | 50 to 75 mg/kg/dose PO or rectally (maximum dose of 1.5 g) |
| Adults | 1 to 2 g PO or rectally |

**Midazolam (Versed)**

| Age | Dose |
|---|---|
| Children | 0.5 to 0.75 mg/kg PO (maximum dose of 15 mg) |

**Diazepam (Valium)**

| Age | Dose |
|---|---|
| Children | 0.2 to 0.3 mg/kg PO (maximum dose of 10 mg) |
| Adults | 10 mg |

**Lorazepam (Ativan)**

| Age | Dose |
|---|---|
| Infants and children | 0.05 kg/kg/dose PO (maximum dose of 2 mg) |

| Adults | 2 mg PO (maximum dose of 4 mg) |

## Morphine sulfate

| Age | Dose |
| --- | --- |
| Infants and children | 0.2 to 0.5 mg/kg |

## Pentobarbital sodium (Nembutal)

In the care of children, pentobarbital sodium may be given by mouth or rectally. Use only in the care of patients older than 6 months.

| Age | Dose |
| --- | --- |
| Children | 2 to 6 mg/kg PO or rectally (maximum dose of 100 mg) |
| Adults | 100 mg PO |

### REVERSAL AGENTS

These medications should always be available when administering sedation.

## Naloxone (Narcan)

This opiate antagonist may reverse the effects of morphine, fentanyl, and meperidine. It may cause nausea and vomiting and cardiocirculatory alterations. The onset of its effect occurs 2 minutes after administration, and the effect lasts 20 to 60 minutes.

| Age | Dose |
| --- | --- |
| Infants and children | 0.005 to 0.01 mg/kg/dose IV every 2 to 3 minutes for maximum of three doses |
|  | Reversal of narcotic overdose may require doses of 0.05 to 0.1 mg/kg |
| Adults | 0.4 to 2 mg IV every 2 to 3 minutes |

## Flumazenil (Mazicon)

This medication may reverse the effects of midazolam, diazepam, and lorazepam. It may cause nausea and vomiting, cardiac arrhythmias, blurred vision, and seizures.

| Age | Dose |
| --- | --- |
| Children heavier than 20 kg | 0.01 mg/kg IV (repeat dose of 0.005 mg/kg IV after 1 minute) |
| Children lighter than 20 kg | 0.2 mg IV (repeat dose of 0.2 mg after 1 minute) |
| Adults | 0.2 mg IV (repeat dose of 0.2 mg at 1-minute intervals, maximum dose of 1 mg) |

### TOPICAL MEDICATIONS

Use topical lidocaine particularly for children undergoing oral sedation. We have found it very useful when inserting an IV line.

## Lidocaine 2.5% and Prilocaine 2.5% (EMLA Cream)

This drug is to be used only on healthy, intact skin. Its side effects include local and minor irritation and itching. Use of this drug is not indicated for patients younger than 1 month or those with a history of allergy to local anesthetics of the amide type. The onset of action occurs within 1 hour of administration. The peak effect occurs within 2 to 3 hours, and the effect disappears 1 to 2 hours after removal of the cream. Apply a thick layer of cream and cover the area with an occlusive dressing. Dose is one half of the 5-gram tube per site.

## *Postprocedural Care*

We monitor and document vital signs, oxygen saturation, and sedation scale scores every 15 minutes (total of four times), then every 30 minutes (total of two times), and then every hour until release of the patient. This monitoring continues until the patient returns to the preprocedural sedation score.

## *Releasing the Patient*

The supervising physician is in charge of releasing the patient. Patients are advised that residual effects from sedation may persist for some time (according to the medication given). Adult patients are advised regarding the seven Ds, as follows:

1. Driving. Do not drive.
2. Dangerous. Do not operate dangerous equipment.
3. Decisions. Do not make important decisions.
4. Drink. Do not drink alcoholic beverages.
5. Diet. After sedation, eat a light diet and then resume normal diet on the following day.
6. Dizziness. Watch out for dizziness.
7. Discuss. Ask your physician any questions you may have.

Our postsedation guidelines for children are as follows:

1. Provide a safe environment for your child. Keep your child inside and under the supervision of an adult. The child needs to be safely secure in the car on the trip home.
2. Your child may remain sleepy for several hours after the procedure. You should be able to wake your child up by calling his or her name and touching him or her. The child may drift back to sleep.
3. Give only clear liquids for the first 2 hours after the procedure. Resume normal diet once the child is fully awake.
4. Your child should be completely recovered from the medication in 4 to 8 hours.
5. Call _____ at the Department of Radiology if you have any questions or concerns.

# 7  What Study to Order

## Brain

Stroke
1. Diffusion-weighted magnetic resonance imaging (MRI), if normal perform contrast-enhanced MRI.
2. If hemorrhage is suspected, noncontrast computed tomography (CT) may be helpful.

Acute headache
1. Noncontrast CT to rule out subarachnoid hemorrhage and hydrocephalus.

Chronic headaches
1. MRI with contrast.

Seizures
1. Pre- and postcontrast CT is still a good place to start, especially for adults, to rule out hemorrhage and tumors.
2. MRI is ideal for intractable seizures, partial complex seizures, and temporal lobe resection.

Hemorrhage
1. Noncontrast CT.
2. Pre- and postcontrast MRI for atypical hemorrhage.
3. Portable ultrasound scan for premature babies.

Tumors
1. Contrast-enhanced MRI for both primary and secondary tumors.

Trauma
1. Noncontrast CT.
2. Noncontrast MRI may be used for patients who do not improve as expected or for those with a clinical deficit not explained with CT findings. MRI is helpful to date injuries in instances of child abuse.
3. Plain films may be used to document fractures in special cases (e.g., child abuse), because CT may miss fractures oriented in the same plane as slices.

Arteriovenous malformation or aneurysm
1. Catheter angiography is the standard, but screening may be performed with magnetic resonance angiography (MRA).

Extracranial carotid artery disease
1. Doppler sonography is a good screening method.
2. MRA is another good screening method, or it may be used to examine patients who cannot tolerate conventional angiography. The results of MRA should be correlated with those obtained at Doppler sonography.
3. Catheter angiography continues to be the standard.

| | |
|---|---|
| Vasculitis | 1. Catheter angiography. |
| Dementia | 1. Noncontrast MRI generally is sufficient. |
| Hydrocephalus | 1. MRI is an ideal initial study (noncontrast-enhanced for children, contrast-enhanced for adults). |
| | 2. Noncontrast CT is well-suited for follow-up examinations. |
| Vertigo and dizziness | 1. Contrast-enhanced MRI is an ideal imaging method for suspected disorders of the cerebellum, brainstem, and internal auditory canals. |
| | 2. MRA may be needed. |
| Cranial nerve palsy | 1. Contrast-enhanced MRI. |
| Congenital anomalies | 1. Noncontrast MRI. |
| Pituitary disorders | 1. Contrast-enhanced MRI is better than contrast-enhanced CT for intrapituitary lesions, but MRI is much better for evaluation of adjacent cavernous sinuses and suprasellar spaces. |
| Brain death | 1. Bedside radionuclide scan. |

## Spine

| | |
|---|---|
| Degenerative disorders | 1. Noncontrast CT and MRI are probably equivalent; if symptoms referable to conus medullaris are present, MRI is ideal. |
| | 2. Contrast-enhanced MRI is the method of choice to examine the spine postoperatively. |
| | 3. Myelography may be indicated when CT and MRI do not provide adequate information. |
| Infections | 1. Contrast-enhanced MRI. |
| Congenital anomalies | 1. Noncontrast MRI. |
| Scoliosis | 1. MRI (contrast may be needed if tumor is responsible). |
| Tumors | 1. Contrast-enhanced MRI is ideal for screening of cord compression caused by metastases and to evaluate spinal cord tumors. |
| Trauma | 1. Use plain films as the initial study and to assess stability. |
| | 2. Noncontrast CT. |
| | 3. Noncontrast MRI for suspected cord injuries. |
| Inflammation | 1. Contrast-enhanced MRI. |
| Vascular disorders | 1. Contrast-enhanced MRI. |
| Brachial plexopathy | 1. Contrast-enhanced MRI. |

## Paranasal Sinuses

| | |
|---|---|
| Infection | 1. Noncontrast CT. |
| | 2. Contrast-enhanced CT or MRI when intracranial extension is suspected. |

| Trauma | 1. Noncontrast CT. |
| Tumors | 1. Contrast-enhanced MRI and CT. |

# *Orbits*

| Trauma | 1. Noncontrast CT. |
| | 2. Plain films or CT may be used to evaluate foreign bodies. |
| Infection or inflammation | 1. Contrast-enhanced CT is the ideal screening study. |
| | 2. Contrast-enhanced MRI is helpful for intracranial extension. |
| Tumors | 1. Contrast-enhanced CT is good for tumors confined to the globe, especially in children; contrast-enhanced MRI is ideal for intraocular tumors (melanoma) in adults. |
| | 2. Contrast-enhanced MRI is ideal for extension outside the globe. |
| Congenital anomalies | 1. Noncontrast CT is a good initial study, but noncontrast MRI may help in further characterizing the lesion. |

# *Neck*

| Tumor | 1. Contrast-enhanced CT to evaluate laryngeal tumors. |
| | 2. Contrast-enhanced MRI or CT or both to evaluate tumors between the palate and hyoid bone. |
| | 3. Contrast-enhanced MRI or CT or both to evaluate tumors above the palate. |
| Infection | 1. Contrast-enhanced CT (remember that the airway may be compromised). |
| Congenital anomalies | 1. Contrast-enhanced CT is a good initial study, but MRI may be needed. |

*Part II*
# *IMAGING FUNDAMENTALS*

# 8 Trauma

## Skull Fracture

### KEY FACTS

- Linear fractures or sutural diastases with no underlying brain injury are generally not clinically significant; formation of leptomeningeal cysts (growing fracture) is very rare.
- Fractures through the base of skull or paranasal sinuses may produce pneumocephalus.
- Fracture through the base of skull may give origin to gas in the temporomandibular joint.
- In a depressed fracture, fragments are displaced by more than 0.5 cm; most depressed fractures have underlying contusions, and contrecoup injuries are present in 30% of patients.
- Most depressed fractures are considered open and require débridement.
- Most skull fractures have no underlying brain injuries, and most severe brain injuries have no skull fractures. Plain radiographs are not useful in suspected cerebral trauma.

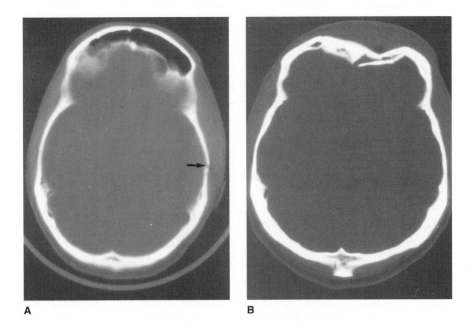

**FIGURE 8-1** (A) Axial computed tomographic (CT) scan shows linear nondisplaced fracture (*arrow*) of the left temporal squama. (B) Axial CT scan demonstrates comminuted and depressed fracture of the frontal sinus.

## Suggested Reading

Masters SJ, McClean PM, Arcarese JS, et al. Skull x-ray examinations after head trauma. *N Engl J Med* 1987;316:84.

# *Epidural Hematoma*

## KEY FACTS

- About 70% to 75% of instances of epidural hematoma occur in the temporoparietal region and are caused by laceration of the middle meningeal artery.

- Computed tomography (CT) helps identify underlying fracture in 85% to 95% of instances of epidural hematoma.

- A lucid interval is seen among only 50% of patients; the overall mortality rate is 5%; delayed enlargement of the hematoma occurs in 10% to 30% of instances.

- In children, epidural hematomas may arise from laceration of venous sinuses.

- A venous sinus origin should be suspected when the hematoma abuts both sides of the tentorium.

- Approximately 95% of epidural hematomas are supratentorial and unilateral.

- 50% to 75% of victims of severe head trauma have an epidural hematoma.

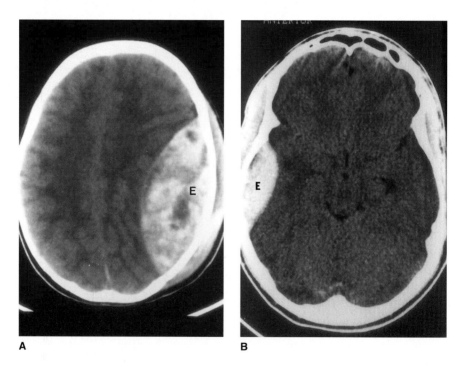

**A**    **B**

**FIGURE 8-2**    **(A)** Axial CT shows large left epidural hematoma (E) in a child. Mixed areas of attenuation are not unusual in childhood epidural hematomas. **(B)** Axial CT in an adult shows right temporal epidural hematoma (E) with typical biconvex configuration.

## Suggested Reading

Osborn AG. Craniocerebral trauma. In: *Diagnostic neuroradiology.* St. Louis: Mosby, 1994:204.

# *Subdural Hematoma and Hygroma*

## KEY FACTS

- About 95% of subdural hematomas occur in frontoparietal regions and are caused by tearing of bridging veins.

- About 10% to 15% of subdural hematomas are bilateral; an interhemispheric location in children suggests abuse.

- The overall mortality rate for patients with subdural hematomas is 60% to 90%.

- Subdural hematomas, CT findings: acute hematomas (<3 days) are crescentic and hyperdense; isodensity occurs between a few days to 3 weeks; chronic (hypodense) hematomas are older than 3 weeks.

- Both isodense and hypodense subdural hematomas may have membrane enhancement.

- Visualization of small subdural hematomas requires the use of intermediate CT window settings (width, 250; level, 40). All trauma cases ideally should be imaged at three levels (bone, intermediate, soft tissue).

- Cerebral contusions are seen in 50% of patients with subdural hematomas.

- Subdural hematomas are found in 10% to 20% of severe head trauma victims.

- Hygromas are collections of nonbloody cerebrospinal fluid (CSF) in the subdural space caused by a tear in the arachnoid membrane. Most occur among older persons.

*(continued)*

## Subdural Hematoma and Hygroma (Continued)

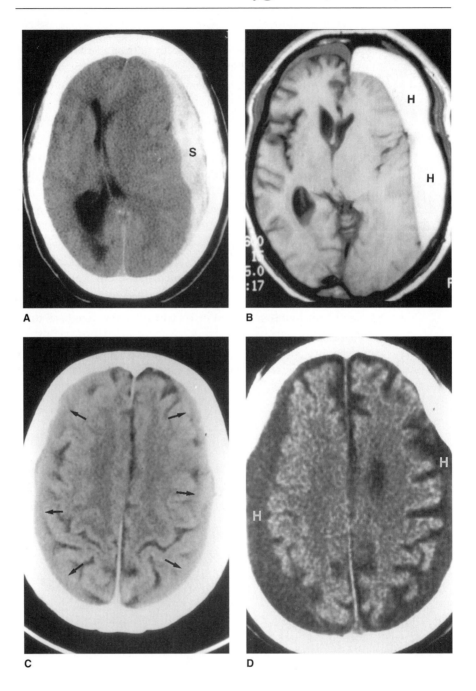

**F I G U R E   8 - 3**   **(A)** Axial CT scan shows left hemispheric acute subdural hematoma (*S*). There is midline shift to the right with dilatation of the right lateral ventricle caused by obstruction of its foramen of Monro. **(B)** Magnetic resonance (MR) T1-weighted image shows large left hemispheric subdural hematoma (*H*). The brightness is probably caused by the presence of methemoglobin. There is a small right frontal subdural hematoma. Midline shift to the right is present. **(C)** Axial CT scan shows bilateral isodense subdural hematomas (*arrows*). **(D)** Axial CT scan shows bilateral extraaxial low-density collections (*H*) that could be either subdural hygromas or chronic subdural hematomas.

## Suggested Reading

Gentry LR. Imaging of closed head injury. *Radiology* 1994;191:1.

# *Diffuse Axonal Injury and Intermediary Injuries*

### KEY FACTS

- Most common traumatic brain injury is caused by deceleration and rotation of brain.
- Common locations include the cerebral hemispheres (frontotemporal) at gray-white junctions (50%), basal ganglia, splenium of the corpus callosum, and the dorsal brainstem.
- The overall mortality rate is 50%.
- CT scans are initially normal for 50% to 85% of patients.
- Magnetic resonance imaging (MRI), especially with a short flip angle, is very sensitive for detection of lesions that are edematous and contain minimal amounts of hemorrhage.
- Diffuse axonal injury is the most common cause of a posttraumatic vegetative state.
- Intermediary injuries of the basal ganglia are rare and are caused by shearing of the lenticulostriate perforating vessels. They have a poor prognosis.

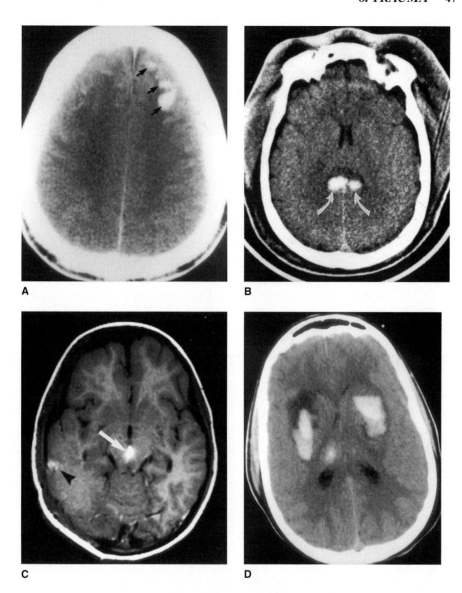

**FIGURE 8-4**    **(A)** Axial CT scan shows left subcortical hemorrhagic shearing injuries (*arrows*). **(B)** Axial CT scan demonstrates hemorrhagic shearing injury (*arrows*) in the splenium of the corpus callosum. **(C)** Axial T1-weighted magnetic resonance (MR) image shows hemorrhagic (methemoglobin) shearing injury (*arrow*) in the midbrain. **(D)** Axial CT scan shows intermediary hemorrhagic shearing injuries in the basal ganglia and right thalamus. These are caused by shearing of the perforating arteries.

## Suggested Reading

Klufas RA, Hsu L, Patel MR, Schwartz RB. Unusual manifestations of head trauma. *Am J Roentgenol* 1996;166:675.

## *Contusions*

### KEY FACTS

- Contusions commonly involve the cortex and are usually hemorrhagic, reflecting the rich vascularity of gray matter.
- They represent approximately 44% of all traumatic brain injuries.
- Contusions commonly involve tips of the frontal and temporal lobes, the undersurface of the frontal lobes, and the dorsolateral midbrain.
- CT scans obtained 24 to 48 hours after injury usually show contusions to be larger because of bleeding and edema, and the contusions may appear to be more numerous than they are.
- Multiple contusions occur in 30% of patients.
- Contusions occur in 5% to 10% of victims of severe head trauma.
- Intraventricular hemorrhage is present in 1% to 5% of patients with cerebral contusions and is caused by tearing of the subependymal veins and choroid plexus.

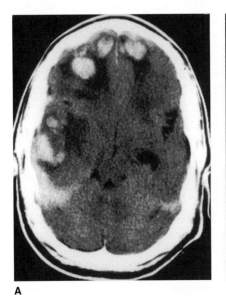
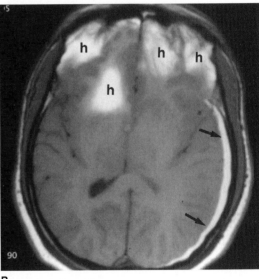

A                                    B

FIGURE 8-5    (A) Axial CT scan shows hemorrhagic contusions in both frontal lobes and in the right temporal lobe. (B) Axial T1-weighted MR image shows bifrontal hemorrhagic (methemoglobin) contusions (*h*) and a left hemispheric subdural hematoma (*arrows*).

### Suggested Reading
Gentry LR. Imaging of closed head injury. *Radiology* 1994;192:1.

# *Traumatic Subarachnoid Hemorrhage*

KEY FACTS

- Seen with most moderate and severe head injuries.
- This type of hemorrhage produces less blood than subarachnoid hemorrhage caused by aneurysm rupture; therefore it almost never induces vasospasm but may produce posttraumatic communicating hydrocephalus.
- CT shows a pseudodelta sign as hyperdense blood layers along the posterior superior sagittal sinus; blood may be seen in the interpeduncular cistern and had to be differentiated from brainstem hematoma or basilar artery aneurysm.
- This type of subarachnoid hemorrhage may arise from extension of superficial brain contusions.
- MRI with fluid-attenuated inversion recovery (FLAIR) images may help to depict subarachnoid hemorrhage not seen on CT scans particularly in a supratentorial location.

*(continued)*

# Traumatic Subarachnoid Hemorrhage (Continued)

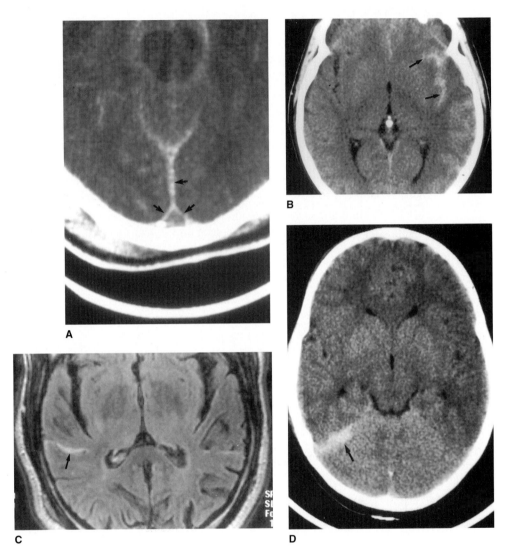

**FIGURE 8-6**   (A) Axial CT scan shows delta sign (*arrows*) caused by subarachnoid blood outlining posterior aspect of the superior sagittal sinus and falx. (B) Axial CT scan shows acute blood in the left Sylvian fissure (*arrows*). (C) Axial FLAIR MR image shows acute collection of blood (*arrow*) in a right temporal sulcus. (D) Axial CT scan shows acute collection of blood (*arrow*) layering on the right side of the tentorium.

## Suggested Reading

Davis JM, Ploetz J, Davis KR, et al. Cranial CT in subarachnoid hemorrhage: relationship between blood detected by CT and lumbar puncture. *J Comput Assist Tomogr* 1989;4:794.

# Child Abuse

## KEY FACTS

- Brain injury is the leading cause of death due to child abuse and is present in as many as 40% of all instances.
- Brain injury due to child abuse is more commonly seen among children younger than 2 years and premature and sick infants.
- Subdural hematomas (particularly of different ages) are the most common intracranial injury and are most often seen along the interhemispheric fissure; they also may be present in different stages of blood breakdown.
- Other imaging features in child abuse include complex (often bilateral) skull fractures, contusions, and shearing injuries.
- Infarctions may be hemispheric because of dissection of the cervical or supraclinoid internal carotid artery.
- Diffuse cerebral edema is more common among young infants than older children.
- MRI is better than CT in depicting and dating injuries of child abuse.

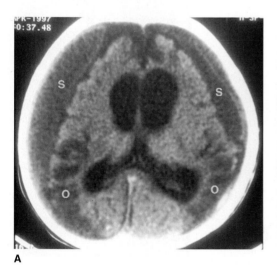 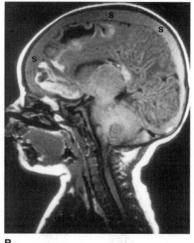

**A**          **B**

**FIGURE 8-7**    (A) Axial CT scan shows bilateral subdural hematomas containing mixed density, which suggests bleeding at different points in time. There are chronic occipital (*o*) contusions. (B) Parasagittal T1-weighted MR image shows a hemispheric subdural hematoma (*S*) and frontal hemorrhagic contusions.

## Suggested Reading

Pettiti N, Williams DW. CT and MR imaging of nonaccidental pediatric head trauma. *Acad Radiol* 1998;5:215.

# *Pneumocephalus*

## KEY FACTS

- Pneumocephalus is defined as the presence of air in any intracranial compartment.
- Most instances of pneumocephalus are caused by trauma (fracture of the frontal sinus) and surgical intervention; infection with gas-producing organisms occasionally may be responsible.
- Most instances resolve spontaneously.
- Tension pneumocephalus has high pressure, exerts a mass effect, results in symptoms, and has to be evacuated.
- Tension pneumocephali are large and occur in approximately 8% of patients with fractures of the base of skull.

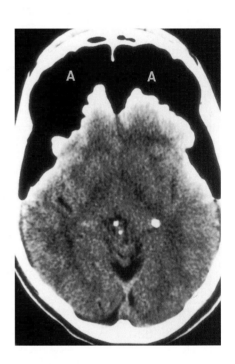

**FIGURE 8-8**
Axial CT section shows large bifrontal tension pneumocephalus (*A*) compressing the brain. The patient had undergone a transphenoid pituitary operation.

## Suggested Reading

Gean AD. Pneumocephalus. In: *Imaging of head trauma.* New York: Raven Press, 1994,135.

# *Arterial Dissection*

### KEY FACTS

- Hematoma is located between the media and adventitia and may create a false arterial lumen between these two layers.

- Patients present with sudden neck pain, Horner's syndrome, or stroke.

- Dissections commonly are located just above the common carotid artery bifurcation and immediate supraclinoid internal carotid artery (ICA).

- When the vertebral artery is involved, it is usually at the level of the axis, base of the skull, and the sixth cervical vertebra (where it enters the foramina transversarium).

- Causes of nontraumatic dissection include fibromuscular dysplasia, hypertension, migraine, use of oral contraceptives, collagen vascular disorders, and pharyngeal infections.

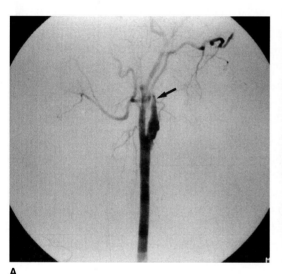
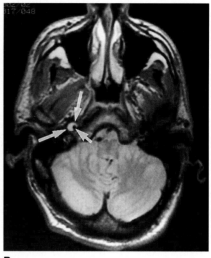

**A**  **B**

**FIGURE 8-9**    **(A)** Lateral digital subtraction view from catheter angiogram shows that the internal carotid artery terminates in a flame-like manner (*arrow*) suggesting a dissection. **(B)** Axial proton density MR image shows hyperintensity (*long arrows*) surrounding the lumen (flow void, *shorter arrow*) indicating mural hematoma in the dissection.

### Suggested Reading

Klufas RA, Hsu L, Barnes PD, Patel MR, Schwartz RE. Dissection of the carotid and vertebral arteries: imaging with MR angiography. *Am J Roentgenol* 1995;164:673.

# 9 Stroke

## Acute (<24 Hours) Middle Cerebral Artery Infarction, CT

KEY FACTS

- Cerebral infarctions are the third most common cause of death in the United States; the mortality rate with each episode varies between 15% and 35%.
- Emboli originating from atherosclerosis of the common and internal carotid arteries are the most common cause of middle cerebral artery occlusion.
- 75% of all cerebral infarctions involve the territory of the middle cerebral artery.
- About 50% to 60% of patients with a middle cerebral artery infarction have normal computed tomographic scans during the initial 12 hours.
- The importance of computed tomography (CT) is in establishing the presence or absence of hemorrhage and therefore prescribing thrombolytic or conservative treatment.
- Early signs (0 to 24 hours) include hyperdense middle cerebral artery on plain CT scan (25% to 50%), disappearing lentiform nucleus, and loss of insular cortex.

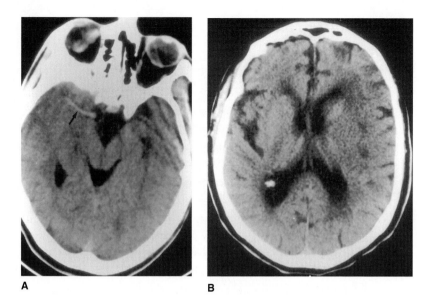

**FIGURE 9-1**   **(A)** Axial CT scan shows a hyperdense right middle cerebral artery (*arrow*). **(B)** Axial CT scan shows subtle low density area effacing the left lentiform nucleus and thalamus.

## Suggested Reading

von Kummer R, Allen KL, Holle R, et al. Acute stroke: usefulness of early CT findings before thrombolytic therapy. *Radiology* 1997;205:327.

# Subacute (2 to 21 Days) Middle Cerebral Artery Infarction, CT

## KEY FACTS

- Hemorrhage (especially in basal ganglia and cortex) occurs among approximately 15% of all patients with middle cerebral artery strokes.
- Mass effect increases during first 3 days, and CT scan shows wedge-shaped area of low density, which involves both gray and white matter.
- CT has a sensitivity of more than 90% in detection of subacute infarction of the middle cerebral artery.
- Gyral enhancement (which may reflect luxury perfusion) begins between 3 and 7 days after ictus and may correlate with a better prognosis than areas of infarction with no gyral enhancement.
- Hemorrhagic transformation may occur 1 to 4 days after onset of infarction.
- Administration of contrast medium may further damage infarcted zone and should be reserved for unclear cases.

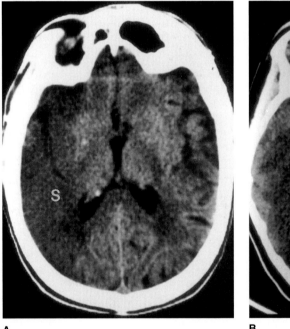
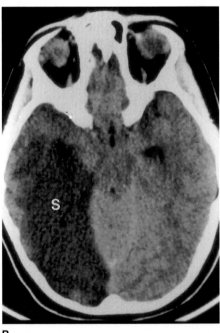

A                              B

**FIGURE 9-2**   **(A)** Axial CT scan at day 3 shows low density (*S*) in the territory of the right middle cerebral artery. Note absence of mass effect. **(B)** CT scan obtained at day 10 shows increased hypodensity (*S*) in infarcted brain.

## Suggested Reading

Weingarten K. Computed tomography of cerebral infarction. *Neuroimaging Clin North Am* 1992;2:409.

# Acute (<24 Hours) Middle Cerebral Artery Infarction, MRI

## KEY FACTS

- About 80% of these infarctions may be identified at magnetic resonance imaging (MRI) during the initial 24 hours.

- Earliest abnormality is intravascular enhancement sign, which may be seen 2 hours after ictus and probably is caused by slow bright intraarterial blood flow.

- Meningeal enhancement overlying infarcted territory is seen in 30% of cases during the first 3 days.

- Cortical edema (hyperintensity, increased thickness, and a blurry gray-white junction) may be seen as early as 3 hours after a stroke, particularly on proton density images.

*(continued)*

## *Acute (<24 Hours) Middle Cerebral Artery Infarction, MRI (Continued)*

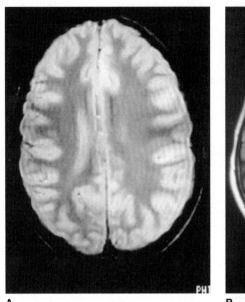

A

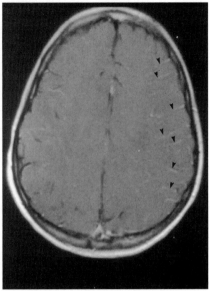

B

**FIGURE 9-3**
**(A)** Axial proton density magnetic resonance (MR) image shows swelling and slight hyperintensity in cortex of left frontoparietal regions. **(B)** In a different case, postcontrast axial T1-weighted MR image shows intravascular enhancement (*arrowheads*) in branches of the left middle cerebral artery. **(C)** Axial diffusion-weighted image (different patient) shows acute infarction (*A*) of the left middle cerebral artery territory.

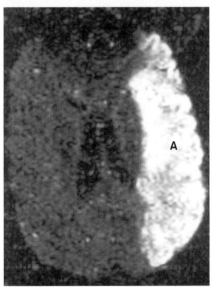

C

### Suggested Reading

Castillo M. Prethrombolysis brain imaging: trends and controversies. *Am J Neuroradiol* 1997;18:1830.

# Subacute Middle Cerebral Artery Infarction, MRI

## KEY FACTS

- Intravascular and meningeal enhancement disappear and are followed by parenchymal (especially cortex) enhancement, which begins 3 to 7 days after ictus and may persist from 1 week to 6 months.
- Stroke becomes markedly hyperintense on proton density and T2-weighted images.
- 75% of all subacute infarctions show parenchymal contrast enhancement.
- Early wallerian degeneration is seen as areas of hypointensity on T2-weighted images along ipsilateral corticospinal tracts.
- Chronic changes of malacia (with loss of volume) occur later, with or without evidence of old blood (hemosiderin).

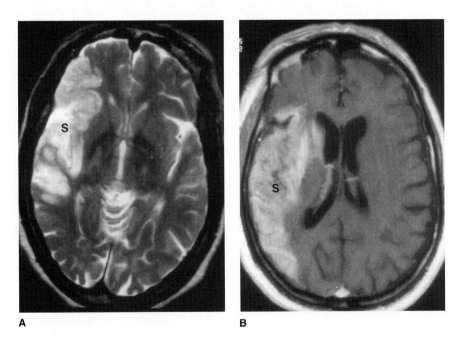

A                                              B

**FIGURE 9-4**    **(A)** Axial T2-weighted MR image shows brightness (*S*) in the territory supplied by the right middle cerebral artery. Note absence of mass effect. **(B)** In a different case, there is marked parenchymal enhancement (*S*) after administration of contrast medium.

## Suggested Reading

Baker LL, Kucharczyk J, Sevick RJ, et al. Recent advances in MR imaging/spectroscopy of cerebral ischemia. *Am J Roentgenol* 1991;156:1133.

## *Acute Anterior and Posterior Cerebral Artery Infarctions*

### KEY FACTS

- Most infarctions of the anterior cerebral artery (ACA) occur in combination with internal carotid artery occlusion; isolated infarctions of the ACA are rare (<1%).
- Most ACA infarctions result in primary vessel disease and not emboli.
- ACA infarctions may be caused by subfalcine herniation and clipping of the ACA under the falx cerebri.
- At imaging the most common sign is hypodensity along the medial cerebral convexity on CT scans or hyperintensity in the same area on T2-weighted MR images. ACA infarction also may produce edema of the corpus callosum secondary to occlusion of short perforating branches.
- Infarction of the posterior cerebral artery (PCA) is the most common infarction after internal and middle cerebral artery infarction. PCA infarction also may be seen with downward transtentorial herniation secondary to compression of the PCA between the temporal lobe and edge of the tentorium.
- Involvement of the medial occipital lobe causes homonymous hemianopsia.
- For all young patients with stroke, consider trauma, drug abuse (cocaine, amphetamines), coagulopathy (sickle cell disease, antiphospholipid syndrome), vasculitis (lupus, granulomatous angiitis), use of oral contraceptives, and use of steroids.

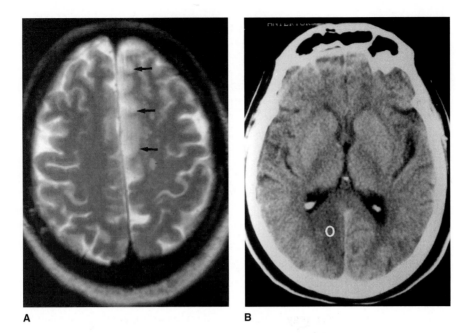

A           B

**FIGURE 9-5**  **(A)** Axial T2-weighted MR image shows increased intensity and thickening of the cortex (*arrows*) in the medial left frontal region. **(B)** Axial CT scan shows hypodensity (*O*) in medial right occipital lobe.

## Suggested Reading

Yuh WTC, Crain MR. Magnetic resonance imaging of acute cerebral ischemia. *Neuroimaging Clin North Am* 1992;2:421.

# *Hemorrhagic Infarction*

### KEY FACTS

- Hemorrhagic infarction is considered as such if blood is identified within 24 hours of the ictus; hemorrhagic transformation of an infarction occurs when blood is identified 2 to 14 days after the ictus.
- Most hemorrhagic infarctions occur as a consequence of ischemic infarction.
- Most hemorrhagic infarctions are caused by sudden reperfusion (lysis of intraarterial clot) of damaged tissues.
- CT scans show hemorrhage in 15% to 50% of patients with large strokes, especially when the middle cerebral artery territory is initially involved.
- At CT, only 5% of all cerebral infarctions are initially hemorrhagic.
- Other types of hemorrhagic infarction include laminar necrosis and venous infarction.
- Although hemorrhagic infarction is assumed to have a worse prognosis than ischemic (pale) infarction, this view has recently been challenged and may not be true.

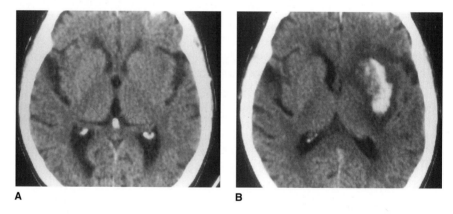

A                                              B

**FIGURE 9-6**    **(A)** Axial CT scan shows subtle hypodensity effacing the left lentiform nucleus (compare with Fig. 9-1B). **(B)** Three days later, there is acute hemorrhage within the area of infarction.

### Suggested Reading
Ebisu T, Tanaka C, Umeda M, et al. Hemorrhagic and nonhemorrhagic stroke: diagnosis with diffusion-weighted and T2-weighted echo-planar MR imaging. *Radiology* 1997;203:823.

# *Wallerian Degeneration*

## KEY FACTS

- Wallerian degeneration generally occurs after cerebral infarction but may be seen with hemorrhage, tumors, trauma, and primary white-matter disease.

- Wallerian degeneration refers to anterograde degeneration of axons and their myelin.

- This condition is rarely seen during the first month after a stroke, but 4 weeks after ictus, a band of hypointensity along the ipsilateral corticospinal tract may be seen on T2-weighted MR images.

- About 2 to 3 months after a stroke, the ipsilateral corticospinal tract becomes hyperintense on T2-weighted MR images, and there is associated atrophy (which may be especially obvious in the affected cerebral peduncle).

- The medial ipsilateral thalamus may show increased T2 signal intensity as the result of middle cerebral artery infarction.

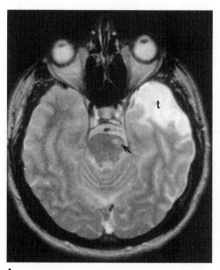 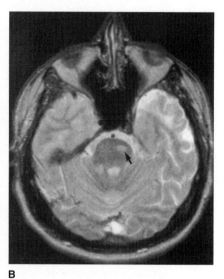

A       B

**FIGURE 9-7** **(A)** Axial CT scan shows old infarction (*t*) in the left temporal lobe. There is high signal intensity (*arrow*) and atrophy of the ipsilateral midbrain. **(B)** High signal intensity (*arrow*) along the corticospinal tract and slight atrophy of the brainstem on that side.

## Suggested Reading

Kuhn MJ, Mikulis DJ, Ayoub DM, et al. Wallerian degeneration after cerebral infarction: evaluation with sequential MR imaging. *Radiology* 1989;172:179.

# *Acute Cerebellar Infarction*

## KEY FACTS

- The posterior inferior cerebellar artery is more commonly involved (and may produce Wallenberg's syndrome), followed by the superior and anterior inferior cerebellar arteries.
- Cerebellar infarction may occur in association with basilar artery occlusion.
- Cerebellar infarction may rapidly lead to death caused by compression of the brainstem and acute obstructive hydrocephalus (caused by compression of the fourth ventricle).
- Upward cerebellar herniation (seen as effacement of quadrigeminal plate cistern) may occur.
- Emergency resection of involved cerebellum may be required as a life-saving measure.

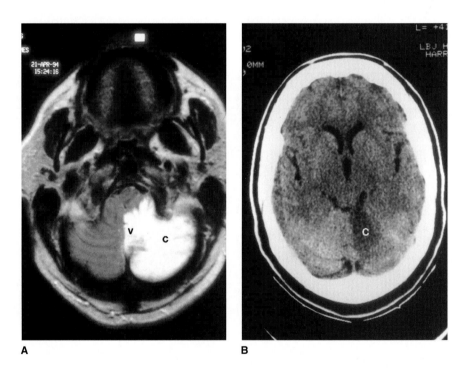

A                                                        B

**FIGURE  9-8**    **(A)** Axial T2-weighted MR image shows hyperintensity in inferior left cerebellar hemisphere (*C*) and vermis (*V*) compatible with infarction in the territory of the left posterior inferior cerebellar artery. **(B)** Axial CT scan of a different patient shows infarction (*C*) in the territory of the left superior cerebellar artery.

## Suggested Reading

Johnson MH, Christman CW. Posterior circulation infarction: anatomy, pathophysiology, and clinical correlation. *Semin Ultrasound CT MR* 1995;16:237.

# *Basilar Artery Occlusion*

KEY FACTS

- Mortality rate is 2.5 times higher than with occlusion of one internal carotid artery.
- Common causes include embolism, atherosclerosis, vascular malformations of base of skull, syphilis, tuberculosis, and fungal meningitis.
- If only the distal part of the basilar artery is occluded, top-of-the-basilar syndrome is produced (infarction of thalami, posterior limb of internal capsules, and midbrain).
- Infarction of the pons may lead to locked-in syndrome (retained consciousness and voluntary eye movement with quadriparesis).
- Because of the high mortality rate associated with basilar artery occlusion, intraarterial thrombolysis may be attempted even though it carries a 30% mortality-morbidity risk.

*(continued)*

## *Basilar Artery Occlusion (Continued)*

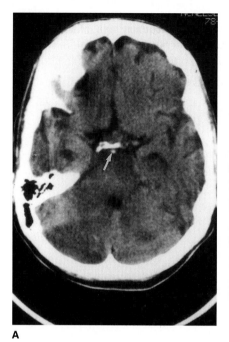

**A**

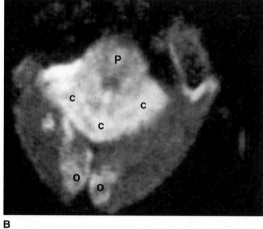

**B**

**FIGURE 9-9**

**(A)** Axial CT scan shows hypodensity
involving the brainstem and cerebellum (right
> left). Note hyperdensity in thrombosed
basilar artery (*arrow*). **(B)** In a different case,
axial diffusion-weighted image shows
hyperintensity in pons (*p*), cerebellum (*c*), and
occipital (*o*) lobes. **(C)** MR angiogram shows
absence of flow in vertebrobasilar system
caused by thrombosis of the basilar artery.

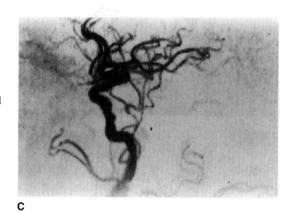

**C**

### Suggested Reading

Castillo M, Falcone S, Naidich TP, et al. Imaging features of acute basilar artery thrombosis. *Neuroradiology* 1994;36:426.

# Generalized Brain Hypoxia or Ischemia

KEY FACTS

- Causes of generalized brain hypoxia or ischemia among adults include trauma, severe hypotension or hypertension, acute irradiation, and venous sinus occlusion. Among children, dehydration, neonatal anoxia, and child abuse are common causes.
- Hypoxia and ischemia involve deep gray nuclei or they cause diffuse edema with effacement of all gray-white borders.
- Generalized hypoxia may give origin to watershed (border zone) infarction or laminar (deep layers of cortex) necrosis (see Laminar Necrosis).
- Contrast enhancement of the cortex may be striking.
- If the patient survives, particularly children, generalized atrophy and multicystic encephalomalacia ensue.

*(continued)*

# Generalized Brain Hypoxia or Ischemia (Continued)

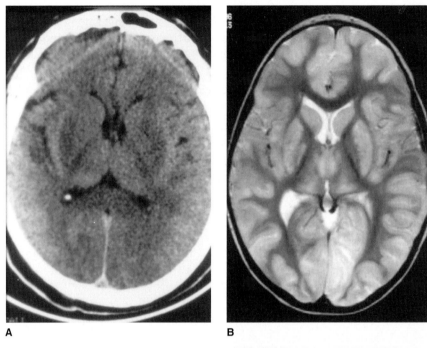

A                                          B

**FIGURE 9-10**
(A) Axial CT scan after cardiac arrest shows areas of hypodensity in lentiform nuclei and posterior limb of the internal capsules. (B) Axial T2-weighted MR image of a child after near-drowning shows hyperintensity in basal ganglia, thalami, and cortex in frontal and temporooccipital regions. (C) In a different patient, axial diffusion-weighted image after cardiac arrest shows hyperintensity in both basal ganglia and temporooccipital regions.

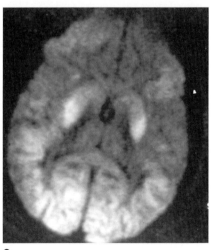

C

## Suggested Reading

Han BK, Twobin RB, De Courten-Myers G, et al. Reversal sign on CT: effect of anoxia/ischemic cerebral injury in children. *Am J Roentgenol* 1990;154:361.

# *Laminar Necrosis*

## KEY FACTS

- Laminar necrosis is ischemic changes in the cortex of the cerebrum and cerebellum.
- Although it is usually caused by generalized brain hypoxia, laminar necrosis may be seen with regional infarction.
- Gray matter layers 3, 5, and 6 are very sensitive to ischemia and are affected in laminar necrosis.
- Usually the watershed zones in the parietooccipitotemporal regions are affected.
- In the acute stage, MR shows cortical enhancement. Areas of hyperintensity in the cortex on noncontrast T1-weighted MR images are seen in the subacute period. Atrophy and hypointense areas in the cortex on T2-weighted MR images are seen in the chronic stage.

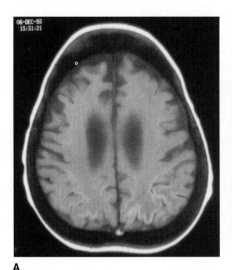 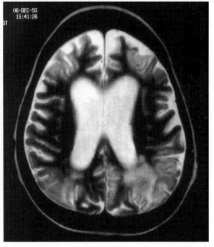

**A**          **B**

**FIGURE 9-11**    **(A)** Axial T1-weighted MR image shows linear cortical hyperintensity in both posterior parietal regions. This could be caused by hemorrhage or lipid-laden macrophages in the infarcted cortex. **(B)** Axial T2-weighted MR image (same patient) shows increased signal intensity in watershed areas. Note thickness of calvarium caused by thalassemia.

## Suggested Reading

Castillo M, Scatliff JH, Kwock L, Green JJ, Suzuki K, Chancellor K. Postmortem MR imaging of lobar cerebral infarction with pathologic and in vivo correlation. *Radiographics* 1996;16:241.

# Superficial Venous Sinus Occlusion

## KEY FACTS

- The superior sagittal and transverse sinuses (particularly the dominant one) are more commonly involved, and occlusion may result in infarction (especially hemorrhagic infarction) in a nonarterial distribution. The sigmoid and cavernous sinuses are less commonly involved.

- Causes among adults include paranasal sinus and mastoid infections, use of oral contraceptives, hypercoagulable states, collagen vascular disorders, pregnancy, malignant disease, and idiopathic causes (25%). Among children paranasal sinus and mastoid infections, meningitis, trauma, and dehydration are common causes.

- The presence of diffuse brain edema and hemorrhage carries a poor prognosis.

- Contrast-enhanced CT may show a "delta sign" caused by filling defect (clot) surrounded by hyperdense venous blood in the superior sagittal sinus.

- Noncontrast MRI shows hyperintensity and lack of flow void in the sinus and dural enhancement. MR venography (two-dimensional time of flight or phase contrast) is useful in confirming the diagnosis.

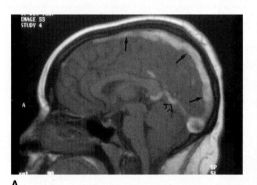 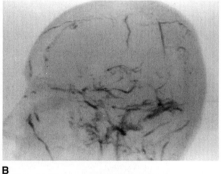

**A**                                                  **B**

**FIGURE 9-12**   (A) Midsagittal T1-weighted MR image shows absence of flow and increased signal intensity in clotted superior sagittal sinus (*arrows*) and straight sinus (*open arrow*). (B) MR venogram (same patient) shows absence of flow in superior sagittal and straight sinuses.

## Suggested Reading

Vogl TJ, Bergman C, Villringer A, Einhaupl K, Lissner J, Felix R. Dural sinus thrombosis: value of venous MR angiography for diagnosis and follow-up. *Am J Roentgenol* 1994;162:1191.

# Deep Venous System Occlusion

## KEY FACTS

- Deep venous system occlusion is less common than occlusion of the dural sinuses or cortical veins.

- It is more common among children than adults.

- Common causes among children include dehydration, paranasal sinus or mastoid infections, trauma (child abuse), and hypercoagulable states.

- Deep gray matter nuclei are involved (which may have hemorrhages), and it may simulate generalized anoxia, both clinically and at imaging.

- Deep venous occlusion is an important cause of bithalamic and midbrain abnormalities.

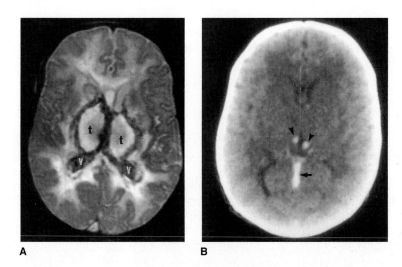

**A**       **B**

**FIGURE 9-13**   **(A)** Axial T2-weighted MR image shows diffuse white matter edema and hemorrhagic infarction of the thalami (*t*). There is also blood (*v*) in the atria of the lateral ventricles. **(B)** In a different case, CT scan shows thrombosis of the internal cerebral veins (*arrowheads*) and straight sinus (*arrow*).

## Suggested Reading

Zimmerman RD, Ernst RJ. Neuroimaging of cerebral venous thrombosis. *Neuroimaging Clin North Am* 1992;2:463.

# *Hypertensive Encephalopathy*

### KEY FACTS

- Hypertensive encephalopathy results from marked acute elevation of blood pressure with escape of fluids and proteins through vessel walls leading to diffuse or focal cerebral edema.

- Common causes include toxemia of pregnancy, renal insufficiency, hemolytic-uremic syndrome, and thrombotic thrombocytopenic purpura.

- In eclampsia most lesions occur in the distribution of the posterior cerebral circulation and are associated with visual disturbances; 90% are reversible, but some produce permanent infarction.

- Most patients show cortical and/or white matter swelling without hemorrhage. The findings are similar to those produced by cyclosporine and tacrolimus.

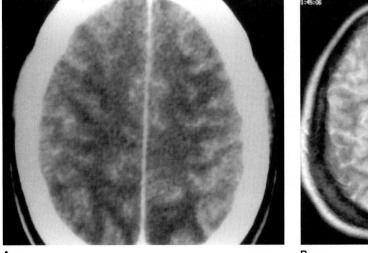 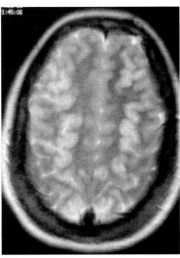

A                                                    B

FIGURE  9-14    (A) In a patient with eclampsia, axial CT scan shows low density in white matter of both hemispheres particularly the parietal regions. **(B)** In a different patient with hypertensive crisis, an axial T2-weighted image shows increased signal intensity and thickening of the gray matter in both hemispheres.

### Suggested Reading

Weingarten K, Barbut D, Filippi C, Zimmerman RD. Acute hypertensive encephalopathy: findings on spin-echo and gradient-echo MR imaging. *Am J Roentgenol* 1994;162:665.

# *Cerebral Vasculitis*

**KEY FACTS**

- Cerebral vasculitis is characterized by inflammation and fibrinoid necrosis of the arterial media and intima, leading to occlusion, infarction, and hemorrhage.
- Common infectious causes include bacterial, tubercular, viral, and fungal meningitis (mainly involving vessels at the base of the brain) and syphilis (mainly involving large-caliber vessels).
- Common noninfectious causes include giant cell arteritis; polyarteritis nodosa; temporal arteritis; granulomatous angiitis (because very small vessels are involved, the angiogram is typically normal); sarcoidosis; collagen vascular disorders (lupus, Wegner's disease, Behçet's disease), primary central nervous system vasculitis, Takayasu's arteritis, and chemical vasculitis (methamphetamine, ergot derivatives).
- Atherosclerosis is not a common cause of vasculitis-like signs and symptoms.
- The mortality rate after hemorrhage caused by vasculitis approaches 50%.

*(continued)*

## *Cerebral Vasculitis (Continued)*

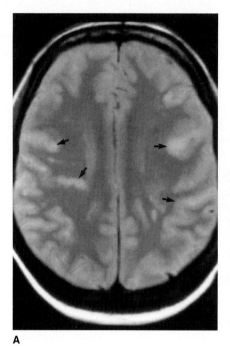

**A**

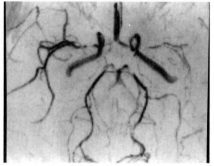

**B**

**FIGURE 9-15**
**(A)** Axial proton-density image shows focal areas of hyperintensity (*arrows*) in superficial white matter and gray matter. **(B)** MR angiogram of the same patient shows multiple areas of narrowing in medium-sized arteries. **(C)** Axial diffusion-weighted image of a different patient with vasculitis shows multiple focal areas of hyperintensity that suggest infarction.

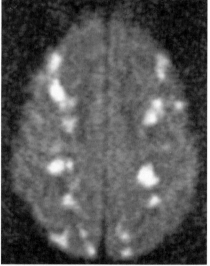

**C**

### Suggested Reading
Harris KG, Tran DD, Sickels WJ, Cornell SH, Yuh WTC. Diagnosing intracranial vasculitis: the roles of MR and angiography. *Am J Neuroradiol* 1994;15:317.

# *Moyamoya*

### KEY FACTS

- Moyamoya disease (also known as idiopathic progressive arteriopathy of childhood) is a primary arterial disorder leading to occlusion of the intracranial internal carotid artery (ICA). It is seen mainly in Japan. Moyamoya syndrome is a radiographic nonspecific finding that is identical to the disease but occurs in association with sickle cell anemia, collagen vascular disorders (Ehlers-Danlos or Marfan's syndrome, homocystinuria), neurofibromatosis type I, Menke's (kinky or steely hair) syndrome, atherosclerosis, and radiation injury.

- At conventional angiography, MRI, or magnetic resonance angiography (MRA), there is occlusion of the supraclinoid ICAs and proliferation of large and irregular perforating vessels and transdiploic collaterals of the external carotid artery (ECA) that supply ischemic regions of the brain.

- Imaging studies show infarction in as many as 80% of patients, particularly children.

- The most common initial presentation of moyamoya disease among adults is intraventricular hemorrhage.

*(continued)*

## *Moyamoya (Continued)*

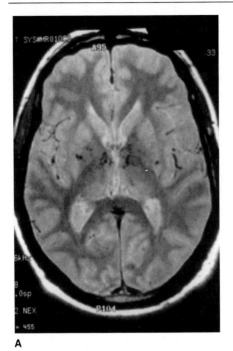

**A**

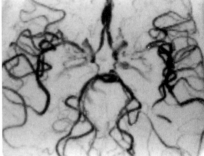

**B**

### FIGURE 9-16

**(A)** Axial proton-density image shows
hypertrophy of perforating arteries supplying
both basal ganglia. **(B)** MR angiogram (same
patient) shows diminished flow and caliber of
both internal carotid and proximal middle
cerebral arteries. **(C)** In a different patient,
axial CT scan shows intraventricular
hemorrhage and dilatation of the ventricles
caused by moyamoya.

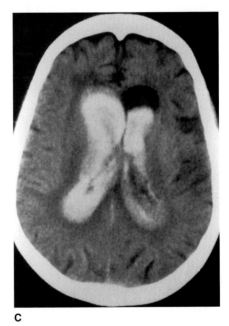

**C**

### Suggested Reading

Moran CJ, Siegel MJ, DeBaun MR. Sickle cell disease: imaging of cerebrovascular complications. *Radiology* 1998;206:311.

# Atherosclerotic Disease of Common Carotid Artery Bifurcation

KEY FACTS

- Chronic injury at zones of turbulent blood flow may lead to a reaction characterized by cellular proliferation, development of fibrofatty plaques, and thrombus formation due to platelet aggregation.
- The most common sources of emboli that cause strokes include atherosclerotic plaques in the ICAs and the heart.
- Vessel diameter has to be reduced by more than 60% by atherosclerosis to produce symptoms.
- According to the North American Symptomatic Carotid Endarterectomy Trial (NASCET), patients with symptomatic narrowing of 70% to 99% of the arterial lumen benefit from surgical treatment.
- According to the Asymptomatic Carotid Atherosclerosis Study (ACAS), men with stenosis of more than 60% of the arterial lumen may benefit from surgical treatment.
- Ulcers can be diagnosed with angiography for only 50% of patients and carry increased risk for cerebral infarction.

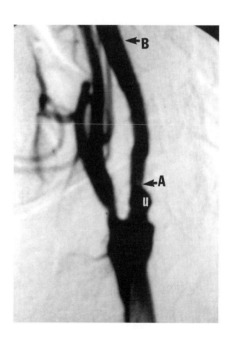

FIGURE 9-17
Lateral angiogram shows 36% stenosis of the proximal internal carotid artery. Calculation according to NASCET criteria are done at level of maximal narrowing (*A*) and normal vessel lumen (*B*) above stenosis. An ulcer (*u*) may be present.

## Suggested Reading

North American Symptomatic Carotid Endarterectomy Trial. Methods, patient characteristics, and progress. *Stroke* 1991;22:711. (Note: Although this article does not appear in the radiology literature, I have cited it here because of its landmark implications.)

# Fibromuscular Dysplasia

## KEY FACTS

- About 90% of patients are women 40 to 60 years of age.

- Fibromuscular dysplasia generally involves the high ICA (95%) or vertebral arteries (at C1-2 level) (15% to 25%) or both; bilateral involvement occurs among 60% to 75% of patients.

- Fibromuscular dysplasia may be associated with intracranial aneurysms (20% to 50%), spontaneous dissection, spontaneous arteriovenous fistulas, and renal artery fibromuscular dysplasia.

- Although fibromuscular dysplasia is generally clinically silent, bruit and focal neurologic deficits may occur.

- The medial form is more common than the subadventitial form.

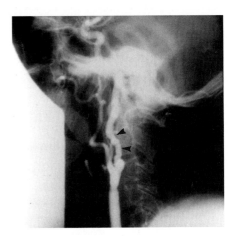

**FIGURE 9-18**
Lateral angiogram shows focal zone of fibromuscular dysplasia (string of beads) (*arrowheads*).

## Suggested Reading

Russo CP, Smoker WRK. Nonatheromatous carotid artery disease. *Neuroimaging Clin North Am* 1996;6:811.

# 10   Nontraumatic Hemorrhage

## *Intracerebral Hemorrhage (Nontraumatic), CT*

### KEY FACTS

- The most common causes of nontraumatic intracerebral hemorrhage include hypertension, ruptured aneurysm or vascular malformation, venous thrombosis, amyloidosis (among patients older than 60 years), collagen vascular disorders, anticoagulation therapies, neoplasia (primary and metastatic), and cocaine use.

- Hypertensive bleeds are more common among men 60 to 80 years of age. Common locations include the basal ganglia (60% to 70%), thalamus (10% to 20%), pons (5% to 10%), dentate nuclei (1% to 5%), and hemispheres (1% to 2%).

- Hypertensive bleeds account for 10% of all strokes and have a 50% mortality rate.

*(continued)*

# *Intracerebral Hemorrhage (Nontraumatic), CT*
## *(Continued)*

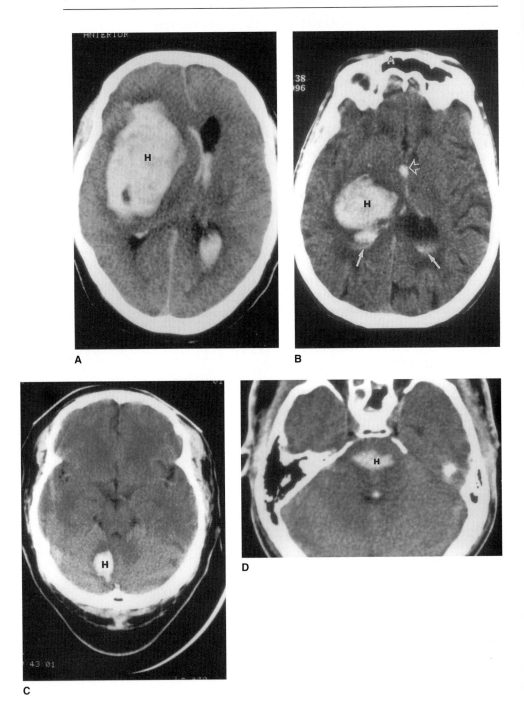

FIGURE 10-1    (A) Axial CT scan shows acute bleeding (*H*) in right lentiform nucleus. There is midline shift to the left and blood in the ventricles. (B) Axial CT scan shows right thalamic hemorrhage (*H*). There is blood in the atria (*arrows*) of the lateral ventricles and third ventricle (*open arrow*). (C) Axial CT scan shows an acute hemorrhage (*H*) in the right dentate nucleus region. (D) Axial CT scan demonstrates a pontine hemorrhage (*H*).

## Suggested Reading

Gokaslan ZL, Narayan RK. Intracranial hemorrhage in the hypertensive patient. *Neuroimaging Clin North Am* 1992;2:171.

# Intracerebral Hemorrhage, MRI

## KEY FACTS

- Oxyhemoglobin (<12 hours) is diamagnetic. Magnetic resonance (MR) appearance reflects water in blood; therefore it is isointense on T1-weighted images and hyperintense on T2-weighted MR images.
- Deoxyhemoglobin (1 to 7 days) is paramagnetic and isointense on T1-weighted MR images, hypointense on T2-weighted or gradient echo images, and starts at the margins of the hematoma.
- Early intracellular methemoglobin (3 to 7 days) is paramagnetic and hyperintense on T1-weighted MR images, hypointense on T2-weighted or gradient echo images, and starts at the margins of the hematoma.
- Late extracellular methemoglobin (after 5 days) is paramagnetic and hyperintense on T1-weighted and T2-weighted MR images and starts at the margins of the hematoma.
- Hemosiderin and ferritin (form after weeks and may remain forever) are paramagnetic and hypointense on T1-weighted, T2-weighted, and gradient echo MR images and start at the margins of a hematoma.
- All findings in the foregoing list are seen at 1.5T field strength; disorganization of different clot stages or contrast enhancement suggests underlying abnormality such as a tumor, vascular malformation, or rebleeding.

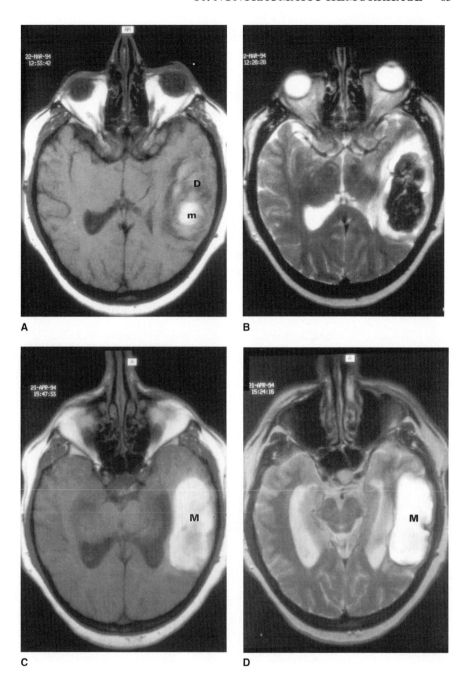

**FIGURE 10-2** **(A)** Axial T1-weighted MR image shows a left temporal hematoma. *m*, intracellular methemoglobin; *D*, deoxyhemoglobin. **(B)** Corresponding T2-weighted image shows that both blood products are hypointense. There is surrounding edema. **(C)** T1-weighted MR image obtained 1 month later shows that the clot is diffusely hyperintense. **(D)** On the corresponding T2-weighted image, the clot is also bright (*M*, extracellular methemoglobin).

## Suggested Reading

Bradley WG. MR appearance of hemorrhage in the brain. *Radiology* 1993;189:15.

# *Periventricular Leukomalacia*

### KEY FACTS

- Occurs among 7% to 22% of premature newborns.
- May occur in utero or during neonatal period and later in life produces spastic diplegia.
- Represents infarction and coagulation necrosis of the watershed zone (between centripetal and centrifugal vascular systems) of the cerebral hemispheres.
- Commonly diagnosed initially by means of ultrasound scan as hyperechogenic regions neighboring the atria of the lateral ventricles; magnetic resonance imaging (MRI) may show periventricular hemorrhage.
- Chronically produces reactive astrocytosis, gliosis, cystic malacia (20%), and atrophy. Findings are more pronounced in vicinity of occipital horns and atria of lateral ventricles.
- Occurs among 50% of babies with intracranial hemorrhage.

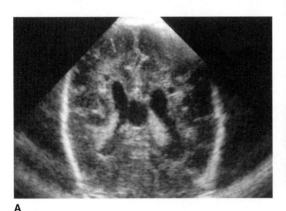

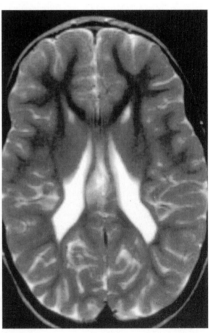

A                                        B

**FIGURE 10-3**    (A) Sonogram shows hyperechogenicity from periventricular white matter, which also contains small cysts. (B) Axial T2-weighted MR image shows the sequelae of periventricular leukomalacia. The posterior white-matter volume is decreased. There is compensatory dilatation of the atria and occipital horns of the lateral ventricles. The outer walls of the ventricles are wavy. In these patients the posterior aspect of the corpus callosum is thin.

### Suggested Reading

Boyer RS. Neuroimaging of premature infants. *Neuroimaging Clin North Am* 1994;4:241.

# *Germinal Matrix Hemorrhage, Grades I and II*

## KEY FACTS

- At 32 weeks' gestation, residual germinal matrix is present at level of caudothalamic notch.

- About 67% of infants born between 28 to 32 weeks' gestation have germinal matrix hemorrhage.

- Grade I implies that the bleeding is confined to the germinal matrix; Grade II implies extension into the adjacent lateral ventricle but without hydrocephalus.

- Grades I and II hemorrhage have good overall prognosis.

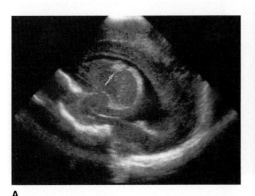 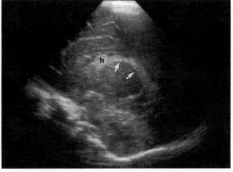

**A**    **B**

**FIGURE 10-4**    **(A)** Parasagittal sonogram shows hemorrhage (*arrow*) confined to the caudothalamic notch. **(B)** Parasagittal sonogram of a different patient shows hemorrhage (*h*) in caudothalamic notch extending into the ventricle (*arrows*). Absence of hydrocephalus makes this a Grade II hemorrhage.

## Suggested Reading

Blankerberg FG, Norbash AM, Lane B, Stevenson DK, Bracci PM, Enzmann DR. Neonatal intracranial ischemia and hemorrhage: diagnosis with US, CT, and MR imaging. *Radiology* 1996;199:253.

# *Germinal Matrix Hemorrhage, Grades III and IV*

KEY FACTS

- Prognosis is usually poor.
- Grade III refers to intraventricular hemorrhage and hydrocephalus.
- Grade IV refers to hemorrhage in the periventricular white matter.
- Grade III bleeding is a continuation of Grade I and II bleeds; however, Grade IV bleeding is probably hemorrhagic infarction caused by compression of deep medullary veins.
- Grade IV hemorrhages have a 90% mortality rate.

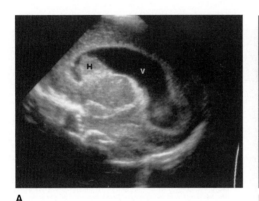 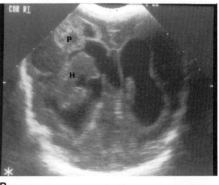

A                                            B

FIGURE 10-5    (A) Parasagittal sonogram shows intraventricular clot (*H*) and dilatation of the lateral ventricle (*V*). The temporal horn is not seen because it is filled with clot. (B) In a Grade IV hemorrhage, there is hydrocephalus, intraventricular clot (*H*), and parenchymal hemorrhage (*P*).

## Suggested Reading

Ghazi-Birry HS, Brown WR, Moody DM, Challa VR, Block SM, Reboussin DM. Human germinal matrix: venous origin of hemorrhage and vascular characteristics. *Am J Neuroradiol* 1997;18:231.

# 11   Aneurysms

## *Anterior Communicating Artery Aneurysm*

### KEY FACTS

- Represent 30% to 35% of intracranial aneurysms.
- Overall incidence of intracranial aneurysms is 2% to 8% of population; risk of bleeding is 2% per year among previously unruptured aneurysms.
- Aneurysms arising from vessels that form the circle of Willis are 90% of all intracranial aneurysms.
- Ruptured aneurysms account for 90% of all spontaneous subarachnoid hemorrhages.
- More than 90% of aneurysm ruptures occur between ages of 30 and 70 years.
- Aneurysms less than 5 mm in diameter are unlikely to rupture (critical size, 5 to 7 mm).
- Ruptured aneurysms of the anterior communicating artery result in hemorrhages in the gyri recti, anterior interhemispheric fissure, septum pellucidum, and frontal horns of the lateral ventricles.
- Rupture of any aneurysm results in hydrocephalus in 10% of patients.
- There is an association between anterior communicating artery aneurysms and the presence of an azygous anterior cerebral artery.

*(continued)*

# *Anterior Communicating Artery Aneurysm*
## *(Continued)*

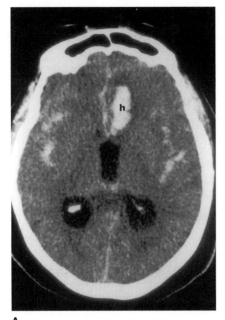

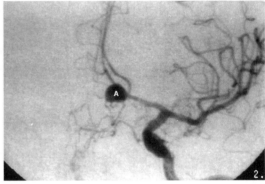

**A**                    **B**

FIGURE 11-1    **(A)** Axial CT scan shows clot (h) in the left gyrus rectus. Blood is
present in the anterior interhemispheric fissure and sylvian fissures.
Hydrocephalus is present. **(B)** Oblique view from catheter angiogram
shows aneurysm in the anterior communicating artery (*A*).

## Suggested Reading

Cognard C, Weill A, Castaing L, Rey A, Moret J. Intracranial berry aneurysms: angiographic
and clinical results after endovascular treatment. *Radiology* 1988;206:499.

Note: General information concerning intracranial aneurysms is discussed throughout the section on
aneurysms. I recommend that it be studied completely so that the reader may have a good overview of
this topic.

# Posterior Communicating Artery Aneurysm

## KEY FACTS

- Represent 30% to 35% of intracranial aneurysms.
- Clinically present with ipsilateral third cranial nerve palsy or subarachnoid hemorrhage.
- Overall, 50% of patients with any ruptured intracranial aneurysm die during the first 30 days that follow the initial hemorrhage.
- Almost all intracranial aneurysms are considered to result from hemodynamic stress, not from a congenital cause (only 2% of all aneurysms are found in children).
- In ruptured posterior communicating artery aneurysm subarachnoid hemorrhage tends to be diffuse but may be concentrated in basilar cisterns.
- Perimesencephalic bleeding may occur without aneurysm rupture and may be caused by tearing of small veins.

*(continued)*

# *Posterior Communicating Artery Aneurysm*
## *(Continued)*

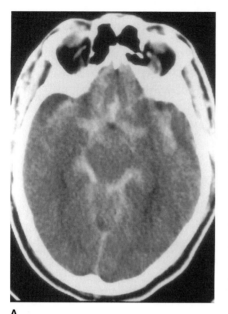

**A**

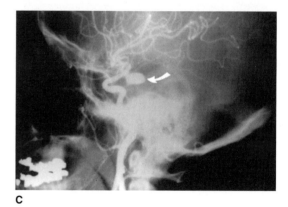

**B**

**FIGURE 11-2**
(**A**) Axial CT scan shows subarachnoid blood in basilar cisterns. (**B**) Axial FLAIR MR image shows subarachnoid hemorrhage (*h*) in basilar cisterns. (**C**) Lateral projection from catheter angiogram confirms the presence of the aneurysm (*arrow*).

**C**

## Suggested Reading

Korogi Y, Takahashi M, Mabuchi N, et al. Intracranial aneurysms: diagnostic accuracy of three-dimensional, Fourier transform, time-of-flight MR angiography. *Radiology* 1994;193:181.

# *Middle Cerebral Artery Bifurcation Aneurysm*

## KEY FACTS

- Represent 20% of intracranial aneurysms.

- Risk for rebleeding from any ruptured intracranial aneurysm is 20% to 50% during the 2 weeks that follow presentation.

- Factors associated with increased risk for intracranial aneurysms include fibromuscular dysplasia, polycystic kidney disease, connective tissue disorders, aortic coarctation, and the presence of intracranial arteriovenous malformation or hypervascular tumors (glioblastoma multiforme, meningioma). Magnetic resonance angiography (MRA) is beneficial in screening these patients.

- MRA helps detect more than 90% of aneurysms 3 mm or greater in diameter, but conventional angiography continues to be the standard.

- Ruptured middle cerebral artery aneurysms result in hemorrhages in the sylvian fissures, frontal opercula, and basilar cisterns.

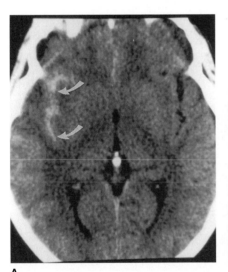

A

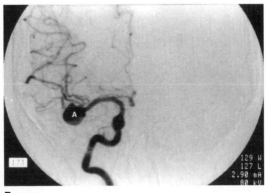

B

FIGURE 11-3    (A) Axial CT scan shows subarachnoid hemorrhage confined mostly to the right sylvian fissure (*arrows*). (B) Frontal view from catheter angiogram shows an aneurysm (*A*) at the bifurcation of the right middle cerebral artery.

## Suggested Reading

Ronkainen A, Puranen MI, Hernesniemi JA, et al. Intracranial aneurysms: MR angiographic screening in 400 asymptomatic individuals with increased familial risk. *Radiology* 1995;195:35.

# *Basilar Artery Tip Aneurysm*

## KEY FACTS

- Represent 5% of intracranial aneurysms. The tip of the basilar artery is the most common location for aneurysms arising from posterior circulation vessels.

- Common causes of all intracranial aneurysms include hemodynamic stress, atherosclerosis, and posttraumatic, mycotic, vasculitis-induced, and metastatic causes.

- Arterial spasm may occur with a ruptured intracranial aneurysm in any location and is generally seen 1 to 3 weeks after ictus; it is an important cause of morbidity (strokes) and mortality.

- Ruptured aneurysms of the basilar artery result in hemorrhage in the basilar cisterns and posterior third ventricle.

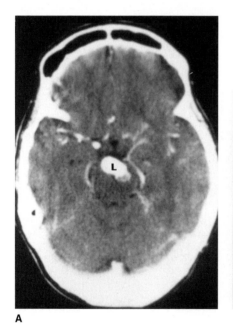

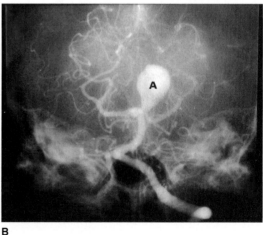

**A**                                    **B**

FIGURE 11-4    (A) Contrast-enhanced axial CT scan shows large aneurysm (*L*) at level of basilar artery tip. (B) Frontal projection from catheter angiogram shows giant aneurysm (*A*) arising from the tip of the basilar artery.

## Suggested Reading

Kallmes DF, Clark HP, Dix JE, et al. Ruptured vertebrobasilar aneurysms: frequency of the nonaneurysmal perimesencephalic pattern on CT scans. *Radiology* 1996;201:657.

# Posterior Inferior Cerebellar Artery Aneurysm

## KEY FACTS

- Represent 1% to 3% of all intracranial aneurysms.
- May present with hemorrhage isolated to posterior fossa or fourth ventricle.
- Both posterior inferior cerebellar arteries (PICAs) have to be studied on all angiograms obtained to rule out an intracranial aneurysm. This examination can be done by means of refluxing contrast medium into the contralateral vertebral artery or injecting each vertebral artery individually.
- Conventional angiography does not demonstrate an intracranial aneurysm in 5% of all patients with spontaneous subarachnoid hemorrhage.

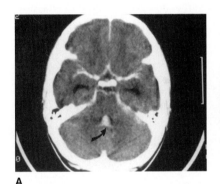 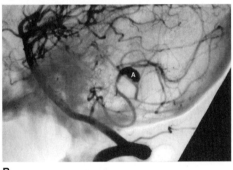

**A**        **B**

**FIGURE 11-5**     **(A)** Axial CT scan shows hemorrhage (*arrow*) inside the fourth ventricle. **(B)** Lateral projection of posterior fossa catheter angiogram shows aneurysm (*A*) arising in the supratonsillar segment of a posterior inferior cerebellar artery.

## Suggested Reading

Urbach H, Meyer B, Cedzich C, Solymosi L. Posterior inferior cerebellar artery aneurysm in the fourth ventricle. *Neuroradiology* 1995;37:267.

# *Multiple Intracranial Aneurysms*

### KEY FACTS

- About 10% to 15% of all intracranial aneurysms are multiple.
- Multiple aneurysms occur most often among women and patients with a family history of aneurysms.
- Helpful signs to determine which aneurysm bled when multiple aneurysms are present include the following: largest, irregular, lobulated (excrescence sign), surrounded by clot or subarachnoid hemorrhage, adjacent vasospasm, aneurysm arising in the anterior communicating artery, and visible extravasation of contrast medium (very rare).
- Incidence of multiple aneurysms: 75% of patients have two aneurysms, 15% of patients have three aneurysms, and 10% of patients have four or more aneurysms.

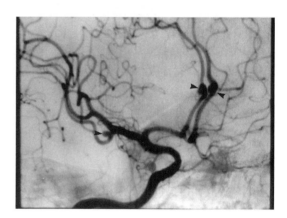

**FIGURE  11-6**
Oblique view from catheter angiogram
showing multiple aneurysms (*arrowheads*).

### Suggested Reading

Wilson FMA, Jaspan T, Holland IM. Multiple cerebral aneurysms: a reappraisal. *Neuroradiology* 1989;31:232.

# *Posttraumatic Aneurysm*

### KEY FACTS

- Account for less than 1% of all intracranial aneurysms.
- When caused by penetrating wounds, posttraumatic aneurysms are commonly associated with gun shots.
- Nonpenetrating injuries produce aneurysms at the base of the skull or distal branches of the anterior cerebral artery as it shears against the undersurface of the falx cerebri.
- Common sites include the intracavernous internal carotid artery (ICA), distal anterior cerebral artery, and distal branches of the middle cerebral artery.

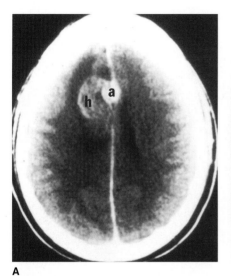
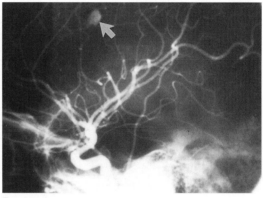

**A**          **B**

FIGURE 11-7    **(A)** CT scan 2 weeks after a head injury shows hematoma (*h*) and a central and enhancing abnormality (*a*). **(B)** Lateral view from angiogram in same patient shows a posttraumatic aneurysm (*arrow*) in the pericallosal artery.

## Suggested Reading

Nakstad P, Nornes H, Hauge HN. Traumatic aneurysms of the pericallosal arteries. *Neuroradiology* 1986;28:225.

# Giant Aneurysm

## KEY FACTS

- Aneurysms measuring more than 2.5 cm in diameter.
- Giant aneurysms rupture less often than smaller aneurysms.
- They mainly produce symptoms by virtue of mass effects (seizures, headaches, focal neurologic deficits, and cranial nerve palsies, especially if located within the cavernous sinus).
- They are more common among middle-aged women.
- The most common sites are the bifurcation of the ICA, intracavernous ICA, and tip of basilar artery.
- Magnetic resonance imaging (MRI) may reveal complex concentric layers of clot along the walls of the arteries.
- These aneurysms grow slowly, and are probably caused by intramural hemorrhages.
- Spontaneous thrombosis occurs in 13% to 20% of instances.

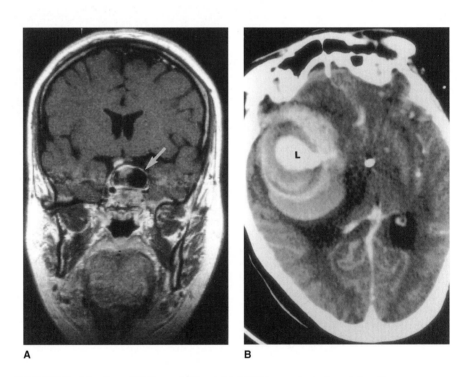

**A**                    **B**

**FIGURE 11-8**    **(A)** Coronal T1-weighted MR image shows large intrasellar aneurysm (*arrow*). **(B)** In a different patient, an axial postcontrast CT scan shows opacification of the lumen (*L*) of a giant aneurysm arising in the bifurcation of the right middle cerebral artery. Note concentric and hyperdense layers of clot along the walls of this aneurysm.

## Suggested Reading

Olsen WL, Brant-Zawadzki M, Hodes J, Norman D, Newton TH. Giant intracranial aneurysms: MR imaging. *Radiology* 1987;163:431.

# 12    Vascular Malformations

## *Arteriovenous Malformation*

KEY FACTS

- Arteriovenous malformations (AVMs) are "congenital" in nature and generally present during middle age (65% of them occur among patients older than 40 years).
- The most common symptoms include hemorrhage (usually parenchymal, 0.5% to 1% of these patients per year), seizures, and headaches.
- Risk for bleeding is 2% to 3% per year, and mortality is approximately 20% to 30% per bleeding episode.
- Factors associated with increased risk for bleeding are deep or periventricular location, intranidal aneurysm, and deep venous drainage.
- Location: more than 80% of AVMs are supratentorial (especially parietal), more than 80% are solitary, and 2% are multiple.
- Multiple AVMs are seen in Osler-Weber-Rendu disease and Wyburn-Mason syndrome.
- The main vascular supply is generally from the internal carotid artery (ICA; pial portion), but large AVMs may recruit external carotid artery (ECA; dural) vessels.
- Computed tomography (CT) shows calcification in 30% of intracranial AVMs.
- AVMs represent 25% of all intracranial vascular malformations.

*(continued)*

## *Arteriovenous Malformation* (Continued)

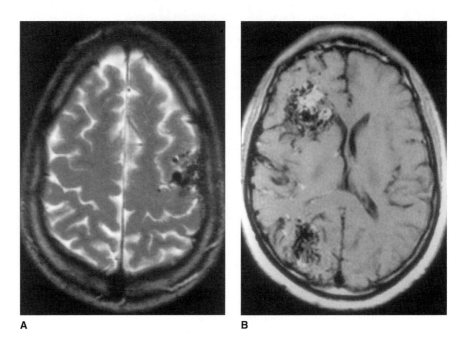

A                                    B

**FIGURE 12-1**    **(A)** T2-weighted MR image shows arteriovenous malformation located in the left medial frontal gyrus. **(B)** Axial T1-weighted MR image of a patient with multiple arteriovenous malformations. There is one malformation in the right frontal lobe and one in the occipitoparietal region.

### Suggested Reading

Edelman RR, Wentz KU, Mattle HP, et al. Intracerebral arteriovenous malformations: evaluations with selective MR angiography and venography. *Radiology* 1989;173:831.

# *Cavernous Angioma*

### KEY FACTS

- Cavernous angioma is a slow-flow low-pressure malformation with no normal intervening brain parenchyma.

- The lesion generally is not visible on conventional angiograms; thus they are angiographically cryptic or occult.

- About 80% of cavernous angiomas are supratentorial, and 15% are multiple (often a familial component is present). These lesions may occur in the presence of venous angiomas.

- Cavernous angioma is the third most common (10%) intracranial vascular malformation.

- The annual risk for bleeding is less than 1%. Bleeding when it occurs tends to be self-limited and clinically not significant; however, risk for bleeding increases after one hemorrhage.

- The most common clinical symptom is seizures; most lesions are asymptomatic.

- CT shows a slightly hyperdense, enhancing focal lesion with calcifications.

- Magnetic resonance imaging (MRI) is the diagnostic method of choice and shows a mulberry lesion surrounded by a rim of hemosiderin.

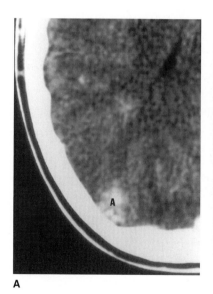 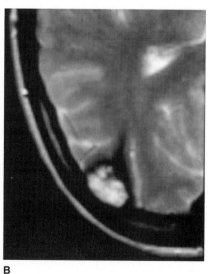

A                                    B

**FIGURE 12-2**    **(A)** Axial noncontrast CT scan shows hyperdense lesion (*A*) in the right parietal region. **(B)** Corresponding T2-weighted MR image shows that the cavernous angioma has a hyperintense center surrounded by a hypointense rim (due to hemosiderin and ferritin deposition).

### Suggested Reading
Horowitz M, Kondziolka D. Multiple familial cavernous malformations evaluated over three generations with MR. *Am J Neuroradiol* 1995;16:1353.

# Developmental Venous Anomaly

## KEY FACTS

- Developmental venous anomaly is the most common cerebrovascular malformation.
- Most anomalies are found incidentally and are asymptomatic; however, they occasionally may present with seizures, headaches, or focal neurologic deficits.
- Hemorrhage is uncommon but may occur with venous angiomas located in the posterior fossa; when a venous angioma bleeds, a coexisting cavernous angioma is usually responsible for the hemorrhage.
- Isolated venous angiomas may be considered an extreme form of a normal variant, because they drain normal brain and are composed of dilated medullary veins that form a large channel that drains into cortical veins (two-thirds of cases) or subependymal veins (one-third of cases).
- More than 65% of venous angiomas are supratentorial, and most occur in the frontal lobes.
- Most venous angiomas are solitary; multiple lesions may be seen in the blue rubber bleb syndrome.
- Venous angiomas may be associated with cavernous angioma; this association presents increased risk for hemorrhage.

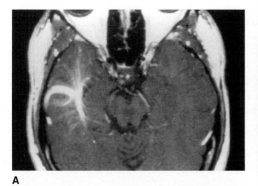

A

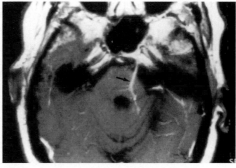

C

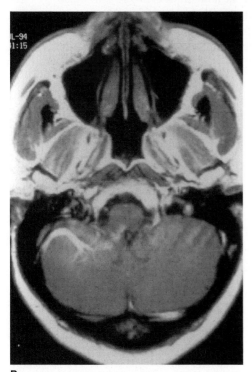

B

**FIGURE 12-3**
(A) Postcontrast axial T1-weighted MR image shows venous angioma in the right temporal lobe. Slow flow results in enhancement of these lesions. (B) Axial postcontrast T1-weighted MR image shows typical venous angioma in the right cerebellar hemisphere. (C) Axial postcontrast T1-weighted MR image (different case) shows an unusual transpontine venous angioma (*arrow*).

## Suggested Reading

Truwit CL. Venous angioma of the brain: history, significance and imaging findings. *Am J Roentgenol* 1992;159:1299.

# *Capillary Telangiectasia*

### KEY FACTS

- Capillary telangiectasia is more common in pons but may occur anywhere in the brain. It is found in 0.4% of the population and is most likely asymptomatic, found incidentally at MRI.

- The lesions generally measure less than 2.0 cm in diameter.

- Histologically the lesions contain capillaries, are surrounded by normal brain, and have no gliosis or hemosiderosis.

- The lesions enhance after contrast administration, are of low signal intensity on gradient echo imaging (probably because of magnetic susceptibility effects caused by oxyhemoglobin), and show no abnormality on precontrast T1-weighted and conventional or fast spin echo T2-weighted images.

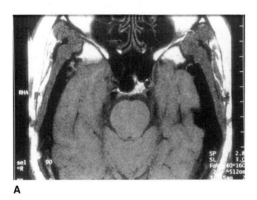

**A**

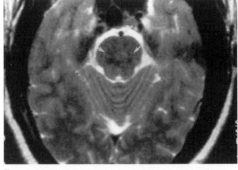

**B**

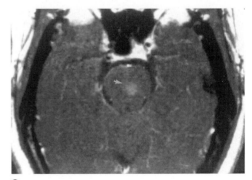

**C**

### FIGURE 12-4

(**A**) Axial noncontrast T1-weighted MR image is normal. (**B**) Corresponding T2-weighted image shows some questionable low signal intensity (*arrows*) in the pons. (**C**) Corresponding postcontrast T1-weighted image shows enhancement in this presumed capillary telangiectasia (*arrow*).

## Suggested Reading

Lee RR, Becher MW, Benson ML, Rigamonti D. Brain capillary telangiectasia: MR imaging appearance and clinicohistopathologic findings. *Radiology* 1997;205:797.

# *Dural Arteriovenous Malformation and Fistula*

## KEY FACTS

- Occlusion of a venous sinus is probably responsible for formation of these lesions.

- Most occur in the cavernous sinuses and in the posterior fossa (near the transverse and sigmoid sinuses).

- Most lesions remain asymptomatic; when symptoms are present, bruit (objective tinnitus), headaches, and bleeding occur.

- Catheter angiography is the diagnostic method of choice.

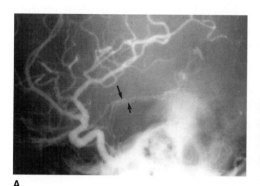
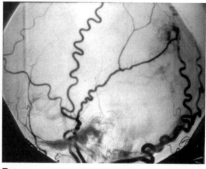

A           B

**FIGURE 12-5** **(A)** Lateral view from catheter angiogram shows a meningeal fistula. The tram track appearance is formed by the draining meningeal vein (*large arrow*) and the smaller feeding meningeal artery (*small arrow*). **(B)** Lateral angiogram (different case) shows fistula to the superior sagittal sinus supplied by the occipital artery and middle and posterior divisions of the superficial temporal artery.

## Suggested Reading

Cognard C, Gobin YP, Pierot L, et al. Cerebral dural arteriovenous fistulas: clinical and angiographic correlation with a revised classification of venous drainage. *Radiology* 1995;194:671.

# *Carotid Artery–Cavernous Sinus Fistula*

KEY FACTS

### Direct (high flow) type:

- These fistulas are a direct communication between the intracavernous ICA and the cavernous sinus.
- Usually seen among young men and constitute nearly 10% of all intracranial vascular malformations.
- Occur secondary to traumatic tear of the ICA or rupture of an intracavernous ICA aneurysm.
- Usually drain into superior ophthalmic vein.
- Present with pulsatile exophthalmos, bruit, conjunctival chemosis, and cranial nerve palsies.
- Treatment is preferably intravascular balloon occlusion with preservation of parent ICA.

### Indirect (low flow) type:

- Less common than the direct type.
- Caused by communication of multiple dural branches from ECA or ICA with cavernous sinus.
- Most occur spontaneously among middle-aged women.
- May be asymptomatic or present with proptosis, conjunctival chemosis, and bruit.

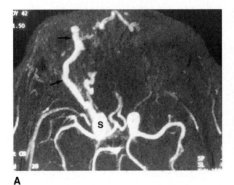 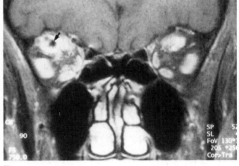

A                                    B

FIGURE 12-6    **(A)** Collapsed view from MR angiogram shows prominent right cavernous sinus (*S*) and very large right superior ophthalmic vein (*arrows*) caused by high-flow fistula between the ipsilateral internal carotid artery and the cavernous sinus. **(B)** Coronal postcontrast fat-suppressed T1-weighted image of a different patient with a high-flow carotid–cavernous sinus fistula. In both orbits, the extraocular muscles are large. The right superior ophthalmic vein is prominent (*arrow*).

## Suggested Reading

Halbach VV, Hieshima GB, Higashida RT, et al. Carotid cavernous fistulae: indications for urgent treatment. *Am J Roentgenol* 1987;149:587.

# Vein of Galen Malformation

## KEY FACTS

- Type 1: Single or multiple choroidal or quadrigeminal feeders empty into vein of Galen; usually presents early in life with congestive heart failure or hydrocephalus.

- Type 2: AVM in midbrain or thalamus with central drainage into vein of Galen; usually presents later in infancy with developmental delay, bruit, seizure, or hemorrhage.

- Type 3: combination of arteriovenous fistula and AVM.

- Intragalenic turbulent flow and distal stenosis probably lead to massive dilatation of the outflow tract and produce vein of Galen aneurysm.

- Occasionally may be thrombosed spontaneously.

- Hydrocephalus is present among 70% of patients and is caused by venous hypertension and mass effect.

- Chronic changes include cerebral atrophy and parenchymal calcifications.

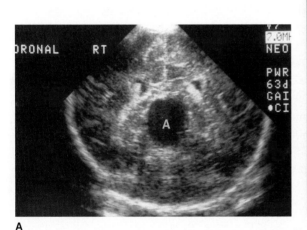 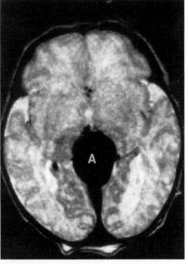

A                                          B

**FIGURE 12-7** (A) Coronal sonogram shows hypoechoic and dilated vein of Galen (*A*). (B) In the same patient, T2-weighted MR image confirms aneurysmal dilatation of the vein of Galen (*A*) in this patient, who had a fistula.

## Suggested Reading

Truwit CL. Embryology of the cerebral vasculature. *Neuroimaging Clin North Am* 1994;4: 663.

# 13 Extraaxial Tumors

## *Meningioma*

### KEY FACTS

- Meningioma is the most common extraaxial tumor among adults, and constitutes 15% of all intracranial tumors among adults.
- Meningioma occurs mainly among middle-aged women (sex hormones may be responsible) and patients with neurofibromatosis type II (especially multiple meningioma).
- Common sites include parasagittal-falcine (50%), sphenoid wing (20%), floor of the anterior cranial fossa (10%), parasellar region (10%), tentorium, and cerebellopontine angle.
- Histologic types are typical (90% to 95%), atypical (3% to 5%), and frankly malignant (1%).
- Classic "hyperostosis" of underlying bone is present in only 5% of cases; typical meningioma may erode bone.
- At magnetic resonance imaging (MRI), a "dural tail" suggests the diagnosis but is not pathognomonic.
- Histologic features cannot be predicted, but bright meningiomas on T2-weighted magnetic resonance (MR) images tend to have more atypical microscopic features.
- Brain edema is present in 60% of cases.

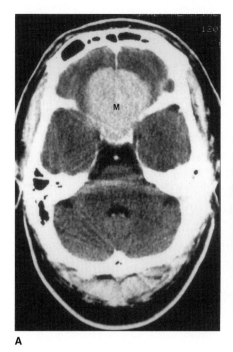

A

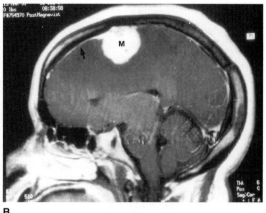

B

FIGURE 13-1 (A) Contrast-enhanced CT scan shows large frontobasal meningioma (*M*). (B) Parasagittal postcontrast T1-weighted MR image shows parafalcine meningioma (*M*) with dural tail (*arrow*) of enhancement. There is surrounding edema.

## Suggested Reading

Buetow MP, Buetow PC, Smirniotopoulos JG. Typical, atypical, and misleading features in meningioma. *Radiographics* 1991;11:1087.

# *Epidermoid*

### KEY FACTS

- Epidermoids arise from intracranial inclusion of epithelial elements during neural tube closure and are 10 times more common than intracranial dermoids.

- These lesions present in early adulthood and grow very slowly.

- The most common locations include the cerebellopontine angle cistern (50%), sella and parasellar areas (10% to 15%), fourth ventricle, and prepontine cistern (all located off the midline).

- May also occur in diploic space of skull (10%), giving rise to a lytic lesion with scalloped sclerotic borders.

- May occur in the middle ear, especially with atresia of the external auditory canal.

- MRI and computed tomography (CT) may not help differentiate epidermoids from arachnoid cysts (diffusion and FLAIR MRI may be helpful in this respect) because of the solid cholesterol that they contain.

- Occasionally, the frond-like surface of epidermoids may be visible at imaging studies.

- Differential diagnosis includes arachnoid cyst, black dermoid, craniopharyngioma, and cysticercosis.

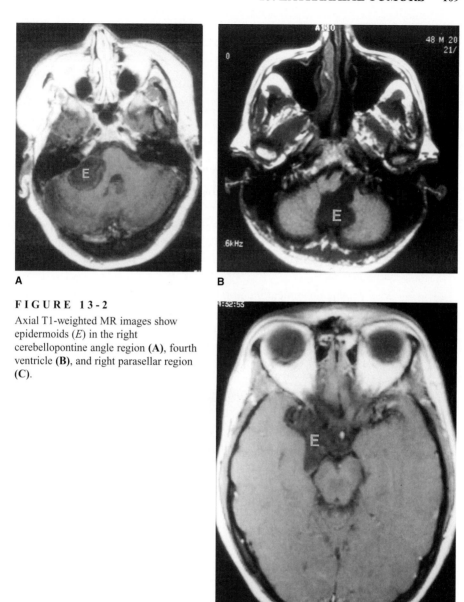

**FIGURE 13-2**
Axial T1-weighted MR images show epidermoids (*E*) in the right cerebellopontine angle region **(A)**, fourth ventricle **(B)**, and right parasellar region **(C)**.

## Suggested Reading

Kallmes DF, Provenzale PM, Cloft HJ, McClendon RE. Typical and atypical MR imaging features of intracranial epidermoid tumors. *Am J Roentgenol* 1997;169:883.

# *Dermoid*

### KEY FACTS

- Dermoids probably arise from intracranial inclusion of ectodermal elements during neural tube closure.
- Rare (<1% of all intracranial tumors), present in early-to-middle adulthood (30 to 50 years) with slight male predominance.
- Most common sites include lumbar spine (associated with spinal dysraphism), parasellar region, floor of the anterior cranial fossa, and posterior fossa.
- Almost all are midline in location (sella, frontobasal region, pineal gland, posterior fossa, anterior fontanelle, and lumbosacral spine) and have the same imaging characteristics as fat because of the liquid cholesterol they contain.
- May produce chemical meningitis if they rupture and spill their contents into cerebrospinal fluid (CSF) spaces.
- Differential diagnosis includes lipoma, craniopharyngioma, bright epidermoid, teratoma, colloid cyst, and pantopaque.

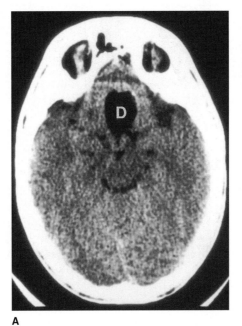
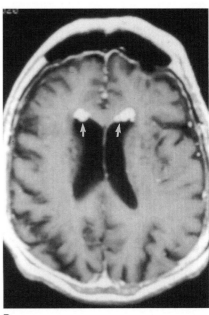

A                                                    B

FIGURE 13-3    (A) Axial CT scan shows dermoid (*D*) in the frontobasal region. (B) In a different patient with a ruptured dermoid, axial T1-weighted MR image shows fat-CSF levels (*arrows*) in the lateral ventricles.

### Suggested Reading
Roeder MB, Bazan C, Jinkins JR. Ruptured spinal dermoid cyst with chemical arachnoiditis and disseminated intracranial lipid droplets. *Neuroradiology* 1995;37:146.

# *Lipoma*

### KEY FACTS

- Lipomas arise from erroneous differentiation of cells (meninx primitiva) that eventually form the subarachnoid space.

- Approximately 85% occur in the midline (50% are pericallosal); other common locations are the quadrigeminal plate, cerebellopontine angle, and suprasellar cisterns.

- Lipomas are generally asymptomatic, but if midline in location, they may be associated with agenesis of the corpus callosum.

- Associated calcification is common.

- Types are tubulonodular (associated with abnormalities of the corpus callosum) and curvilinear (no abnormalities of the corpus callosum).

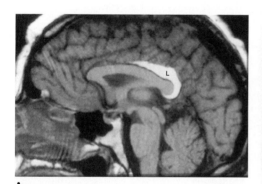
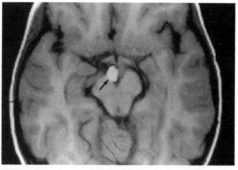

A                                                        B

**FIGURE 13-4**   **(A)** Midsagittal T1-weighted MR image shows curvilinear pericallosal lipoma (*L*). The corpus callosum is normal. **(B)** In a different patient, an axial T1-weighted MR image shows incidental lipoma (*arrow*) in the quadrigeminal plate cistern.

## Suggested Reading

Truwitt CL, Barkovich AJ. Pathogenesis of intracranial lipoma: an MR study in 42 patients. *AJNR Am J Neuroradiol* 1990;11:665.

# Choroid Plexus Tumors

### KEY FACTS

- Choroid plexus tumors represent less than 1% of all intracranial tumors among adults and 2% to 4% of all intracranial tumors among children.
- Most (> 85%) are diagnosed by 5 years of age.
- Papillomas in children more often involve the atria of the lateral ventricles (80%); in adults they are more often found in the fourth ventricle.
- Choroid plexus tumors may cause hydrocephalus because of overproduction of CSF or hemorrhage into subarachnoid space.
- Choroid plexus carcinomas are rare (10% to 20% of all choroid plexus tumors) and are seen almost exclusively among children. Carcinoma should be suspected when there is surrounding edema and invasion of the parenchyma.
- At CT, 20% of choroid plexus papillomas or carcinomas have calcifications.
- About 1% to 2% of all meningiomas arise in the atrium of the lateral ventricles and may invade adjacent brain.
- Other lesions of the choroid plexus are lipoma, xanthogranuloma (usually the result of normal aging), metastasis, lymphoma, meningioma, and cryptococcus.

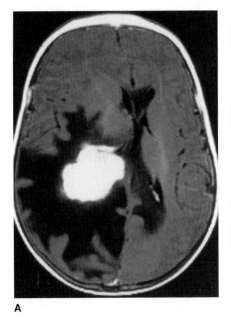 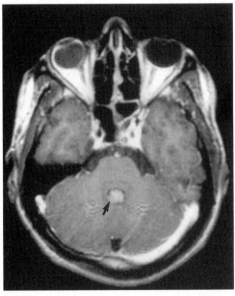

A                 B

**FIGURE 13-5** **(A)** Axial postcontrast T1-weighted MR image shows enhancing mass in the trigone of the right lateral ventricle and surrounding edema. This was a choroid plexus papilloma. **(B)** Axial postcontrast T1-weighted MR image shows small papilloma (*arrow*) in the fourth ventricle.

## Suggested Reading

Coates TL, Hinshaw DB, Peckman N, et al. Pediatric choroid plexus neoplasms: MR, CT, and pathologic correlation. *Radiology* 1989;173:81.

# Craniopharyngioma

KEY FACTS

- Craniopharyngioma is a benign epithelial tumor almost always located in the suprasellar (20%) or suprasellar-sellar (75%) region or is purely intrasellar (<10%).

- Most are found between 4 and 5 years of age; among adults they occur between the fourth and fifth decades of life.

- They present with visual abnormalities (compression of the optic chiasm), endocrine dysfunction (hypothalamus-pituitary compression), or hydrocephalus.

- Histologic types are adamantinomatous (cystic and occurring in children) and papillary (solid and occurring in adults).

- About 85% of these tumors have cysts, 75% measure between 2 and 6 cm, 90% have calcifications, and 90% enhance.

- MR appearance may be extremely variable, but most show low signal intensity on T1-weighted MR images and are bright on T2-weighted MR images.

- Differential diagnosis includes pituitary adenoma, optic chiasm–hypothalamus astrocytoma, dermoid, arachnoid cyst, and aneurysm.

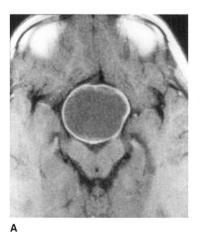 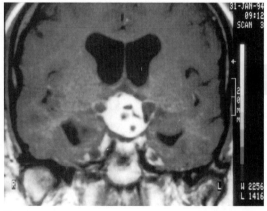

**A**                                    **B**

FIGURE 13-6      (A) Axial postcontrast T1-weighted MR image of a child shows mostly cystic suprasellar craniopharyngioma with peripheral enhancement. (B) Coronal postcontrast T1-weighted MR image of a young adult shows enhancing and mostly solid suprasellar craniopharyngioma. There is hydrocephalus.

## Suggested Reading

Sartoretti-Scheer S, Wichman W, Aguzzi A, Valavanis A. MR differentiation of adamantinous and squamous-papillary craniopharyngiomas. *Am J Neuroradiol* 1997;18:77.

## *Pituitary Adenoma*

### KEY FACTS

- Most (75%) pituitary microadenomas (<10 mm) are endocrinologically active; therefore the diagnosis is a clinical one.
- Most pituitary macroadenomas (>10 mm) are hormonally inactive and present with symptoms related to mass effect (mainly on the optic chiasm, producing bitemporal hemianopsia).
- The most common types of microadenoma include prolactin (27%), growth hormone (13%), corticotropin (10%), and null cell (26%).
- Prolactin-producing adenomas are more common among women and girls; growth hormone–producing adenomas are more common among men and boys.
- Patients with serum prolactin levels greater than 200 ng/mL usually have demonstrable tumor on MR images; a serum prolactin level greater than 1000 ng/mL suggests cavernous sinus invasion.
- About 80% to 90% of microadenomas do not enhance on CT scans or MR images. MRI is slightly superior to CT in the detection of microadenomas; dynamic MRI helps detect an additional 10% of adenomas and is particularly helpful in detection of small ones (Cushing adenomas).
- Pituitary apoplexy is a clinical syndrome (headache, nausea, vomiting, photophobia, nuchal rigidity, vision deficits, and altered consciousness) that may be caused by hemorrhage into the gland.
- Factors predisposing to pituitary hemorrhage are adenoma, radiation, bromocriptine therapy, pregnancy, trauma, anticoagulation, lumbar puncture, and angiography.

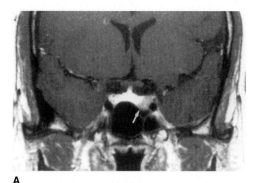

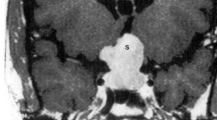

**A**  **B**

**FIGURE 13-7**

**(A)** Coronal postcontrast T1-weighted MR image shows adenoma (*arrow*) in the left lateral wing of the gland. **(B)** Coronal postcontrast T1-weighted MR image shows macroadenoma with typical figure-of-eight shape and suprasellar (*s*) extension. **(C)** Midsagittal noncontrast T1-weighted MR image shows brightness of gland caused by hemorrhage.

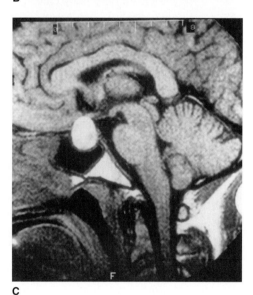

**C**

## Suggested Reading

Bartynski WS, Lin L. Dynamic and conventional spin-echo MR of pituitary microlesions. *Am J Neuroradiol* 1997;18:965.

# *Pineal Gland Tumors*

### KEY FACTS

- Pineal gland tumors represent 1% to 2% of all intracranial tumors among adults and 3% to 8% of all intracranial tumors among children.
- Of the germ cell tumors, germinoma is the most common (50%); most present among men during the second and third decades of life.
- Germinomas may be slightly hyperdense on noncontrast CT scans and of low intensity on T2-weighted MR images, because of a high nuclei-to-cytoplasm ratio; they enhance deeply after administration of contrast medium. Fifty percent of lesions show dissemination in the subarachnoid space at time of diagnosis.
- Teratoma is the second most common primary tumor of the pineal gland.
- Pineal cell tumors (pineocytoma or pineoblastoma) are rare (<15% of pineal tumors), occur among adults, and have no gender predilection.
- Pineoblastomas may be categorized as primitive neuroectodermal tumors; most are found before 10 years of age.
- All pineal tumors may seed the subarachnoid space.
- Other pineal tumors include choriocarcinoma, endodermal sinus tumor, and embryonal cell carcinoma.
- Pineal cysts may have a heterogenous appearance and at times may be indistinguishable from true neoplasms. Most measure between 10 to 15 mm in diameter, occur among more than 5% of the population, and may enhance on delay MR images.
- At CT, the pineal gland shows calcification after 10 years of age.

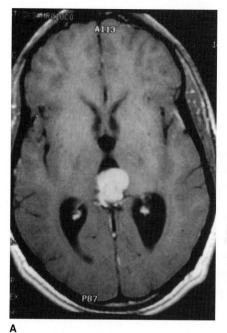

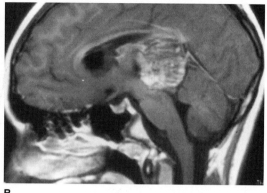

A

B

## FIGURE 13-8

(A) Axial postcontrast T1-weighted MR image shows nonspecific appearance of enhancing pineal germinoma. (B) Midsagittal postcontrast T1-weighted MR image shows large pineal teratoma.

## Suggested Reading

Smirniotopoulos JG, Rushing EJ, Mena H. Pineal region masses: differential diagnosis. *Radiographics* 1992;12:577.

# Colloid Cyst

### KEY FACTS

- Colloid cysts account for less than 1% of intracranial tumors.
- They usually arise in the anterosuperior portion of the third ventricle, possibly from choroid plexus elements, and obstruct the foramina of Monro, producing hydrocephalus.
- Patients present with headache (migraine-like), mental status changes, nausea, and vomiting (particularly severe in the morning).
- Treatment choices include resection, stereotactic aspiration, and ventricular shunting.
- The lesions characteristically are of high signal intensity on T1-weighted MR images and very low signal intensity on T2-weighted MR images, probably because of paramagnetic effects from iron, copper, and magnesium (some authors dispute this).
- At CT the lesions are hyperdense and generally measure 10 to 20 mm in diameter.

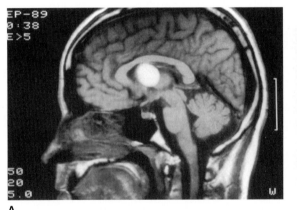 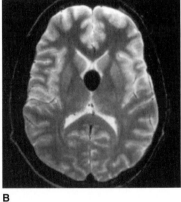

A                                                              B

**FIGURE 13-9**    (A) Noncontrast midsagittal T1-weighted MR image shows large hyperintense colloid cyst. (B) For the same patient, axial T2-weighted MR image shows the cyst to be markedly hypointense.

## Suggested Reading

Maeder PP, Holtas SL, Basibuyuk LN, et al. Colloid cysts of the third ventricle: correlation of MR and CT findings with history and chemical analysis. *Am J Neuroradiol* 1990;11:575.

## *Arachnoid Cyst*

---

KEY FACTS

- Arachnoid cysts account for <1% of intracranial masses, are usually found in children, and are more common among boys.
- Common locations include the sylvian fissure (50%), suprasellar (10%) and quadrigeminal plate cisterns (10%), cerebellopontine angle (5% to 10%) and supracerebellar cisterns (<5%), and cisterna magna (<5%), prepontine cistern, and convexities.
- Histologic subtypes include the leptomeningeal and intraarachnoid types, which cannot be separated on the basis of imaging but probably are not clinically important.
- Arachnoid cysts appear as CSF equivalent masses with all imaging modalities; the main differential diagnosis is epidermoid (distinction may require diffusion MRI or fluid-attenuated inversion recovery (FLAIR) sequences.
- May produce adjacent bone changes (scalloping).
- The only reliable way to assess communication with remainder of CSF spaces is with contrast CT cisternography.

*(continued)*

## *Arachnoid Cyst (Continued)*

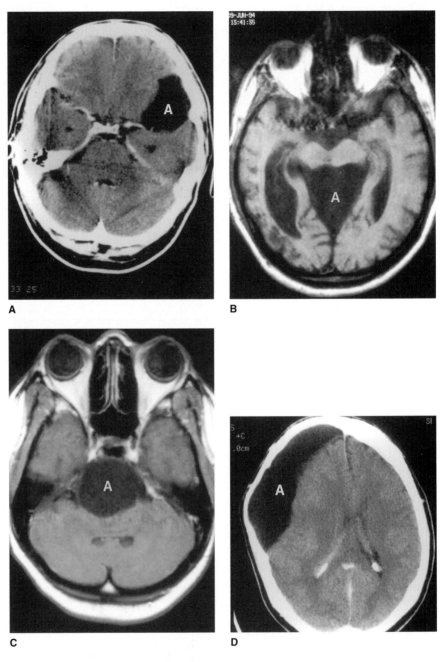

**FIGURE 13-10**  (A) Postcontrast axial CT scan shows arachnoid cyst (*A*) in the left sylvian fissure. (B) Axial T1-weighted MR image shows arachnoid cyst (*A*) in the quadrigeminal plate cistern. (C) Axial postcontrast T1-weighted MR image shows arachnoid cyst (*A*) in the prepontine cistern. (D) Axial CT scan shows arachnoid cyst (*A*) in the right temporofrontal region.

## Suggested Reading

Garcia Santos JM, Martinez Lage J, Gilabert Ubeda A, Capel Aleman A, Climent Oltra V. Arachnoid cysts of the middle cranial fossa: a consideration of their origins based on imaging. *Neuroradiology* 1993;35:355.

# 14 Intraaxial Tumors

## SUPRATENTORIAL TUMORS

### *Astrocytoma (Low Grade)*

KEY FACTS

- Astrocytomas account for 10% to 30% of cerebral gliomas among adults.
- Histologically they are fibrillary (diffuse), and more than 80% eventually show anaplastic transformation.
- The term *astrocytoma*, according to the World Health Organization (WHO) classification, includes grades 1 and 2 of the Kernohan grading system.
- Astrocytoma usually occurs in the cerebral hemispheres of persons 20 to 40 years of age.
- About 10% to 20% of astrocytomas show calcification at computed tomography (CT); all are hyperintense on T2-weighted magnetic resonance (MR) images; contrast enhancement may be absent or mild; edema and hemorrhage are rare.
- The median survival time varies between 2 and 8 years.

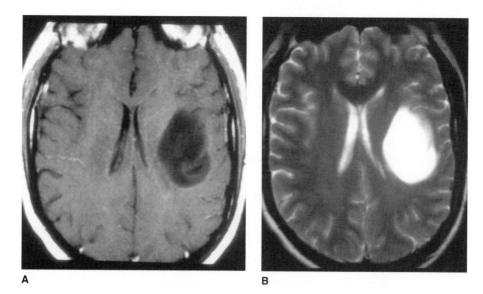

A          B

**FIGURE 14-1**   **(A)** Axial postcontrast T1-weighted MR image shows low-grade nonenhancing astrocytoma in the left temporal region. **(B)** Corresponding T2-weighted image shows well-defined margins and absence of surrounding edema. There is little mass effect.

## Suggested Reading

Castillo M, Scatliff JH, Bouldin TW, Suzuki K. Radiologic-pathologic correlation: intracranial astrocytoma. *Am J Neuroradiol* 1992;13:1609.

# *Anaplastic Astrocytoma*

### KEY FACTS

- Anaplastic astrocytomas account for 30% of cerebral gliomas among adults (40 to 60 years of age).
- Histologically they contain gemistocytes and protoplasmic elements.
- Dissemination through the white matter tracts, ependyma, and subarachnoid space is relatively common.
- The term *anaplastic astrocytoma*, according to the WHO classification, corresponds to grade 3 (malignant) in the Kernohan grading system.
- Anaplastic astrocytoma commonly arises in the white matter of the cerebral hemispheres (frontal, parietal, temporal, and occipital) of persons 40 to 60 years of age.
- Imaging studies show an inhomogeneous mass surrounded by edema and sometimes peripheral or central areas of enhancement.
- The prognosis is poor; the median survival time is 2 years.

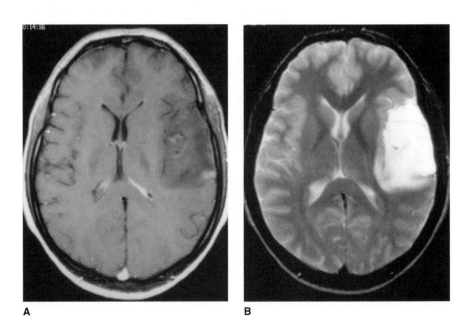

**A**          **B**

### FIGURE 14-2

**(A)** Axial postcontrast T1-weighted MR image shows left insular anaplastic astrocytoma with ill-defined margins and patchy enhancement. There is no obvious necrosis. **(B)** Corresponding T2-weighted image shows the tumor to have ill-defined margins.

### Suggested Reading

Castillo M. Contrast enhancement in primary tumors of the brain and spinal cord. *Neuroimaging Clin North Am* 1994;4:63.

# Glioblastoma Multiforme

## KEY FACTS

- Glioblastoma multiforme accounts for more than 50% of cerebral gliomas among adults (the most common brain tumor among adults).

- Necrosis, neovascularity, and cellular pleomorphism ("multiforme") are typical histologic features.

- The term *glioblastoma multiforme*, according to the WHO classification, corresponds to grade 4 of the Kernohan grading system.

- Most of these tumors arise in white matter of cerebral hemispheres (frontal, temporal, parietal, and corpus callosum) of men after the age of 50 years.

- Imaging studies often reveal typical nodular rim enhancement; edema is generally present, hemorrhage may occur (most common glial cell tumor to bleed), calcifications are rare, and 10% occur in multiple sites.

- The prognosis is very poor; most patients die 8 to 12 months after diagnosis.

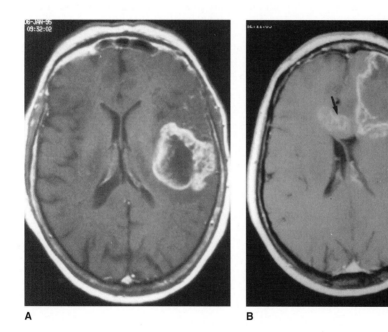

**A**     **B**

**FIGURE 14-3**     **(A)** Axial postcontrast T1-weighted MR image shows glioblastoma multiforme (*GBM*) in the left temporal lobe. Note irregular and thick ring enhancement. There is central necrosis. **(B)** Axial postcontrast T1-weighted MR image shows large and irregular enhancing GBM in the left frontal lobe with extension across the genu of the corpus callosum (*arrow*).

## Suggested Reading

Rees JH, Smirniotopoulos JG, Jones RV, Wong K. Glioblastoma multiforme: radiologic-pathologic correlation. *Radiographics* 1996;16:1413.

# Oligodendroglioma

## KEY FACTS

- Oligodendrogliomas account for less than 5% of cerebral gliomas among adults. They are generally found in the fifth or sixth decades of life and are more common among men.
- About 50% of these tumors are histologically mixed and contain neoplastic astrocytes (called an *oligoastrocytoma,* which is identical to oligodendroglioma on images); growth is very slow.
- More than 85% of oligodendrogliomas are supratentorial.
- They typically involve the subcortical white matter in the frontotemporal regions (but may occur in the temporal and occipital lobes and in the corpus callosum); these tumors are slow growing.
- The most common symptom is seizures.
- Oligodendroglioma is the most common intracranial tumor to calcify (70%). Because of its peripheral location, this tumor may cause scalloping of inner table of skull (17%). Cysts are present in 20% of instances; hemorrhage occurs in 20%; and contrast enhancement is seen in 50%.
- The 5-year survival rate is 75% for pure oligodendroglioma.
- When it arises inside the lateral ventricles, oligodendroglioma may be histologically confused with central neurocytoma.

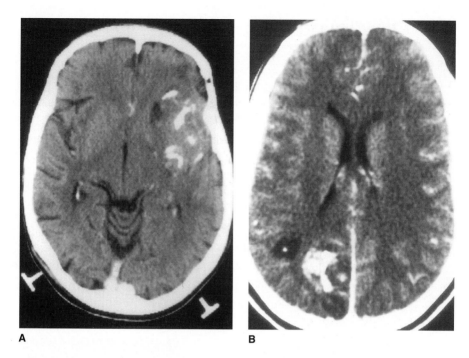

A                                    B

**FIGURE 14-4**     (A) Axial postcontrast CT scan shows an oligodendroglioma with
multiple calcifications in the left frontotemporal region. (B)
Postcontrast CT scan shows heavily calcified oligodendroglioma in the
medial left occipital lobe. There is a tumor cyst lateral to the
calcification.

## Suggested Reading

Tice H, Barnes PD, Gumerova L, Scott RM, Tarbell NJ. Pediatric and adolescent oligodendrogliomas. *Am J Neuroradiol* 1993;14:1293.

# Ependymoma

### KEY FACTS

- Ependymomas account for 2% to 6% of intracranial gliomas. Most often they are found in the first (peak, 5 years) and second decades of life, but they also occur among adults (peak, 40 years).
- Common locations are, among children, the fourth ventricle in 60% of instances (third most common pediatric brain tumor) and, among adults, the cerebral hemispheres (30% to 40% of all ependymomas).
- About 50% to 80% of supratentorial ependymomas are parenchymal (arise from ependymal cell rests) and are located in the frontoparietal regions.
- CT shows calcification in 50% and cysts and edema in 50% of instances.
- The overall 5-year survival rate is approximately 50%.
- Subependymoma is a variant of ependymoma. It is more common among adults. Most of these tumors are subclinical and occur in the fourth ventricle.

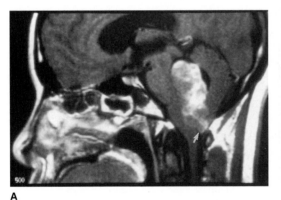
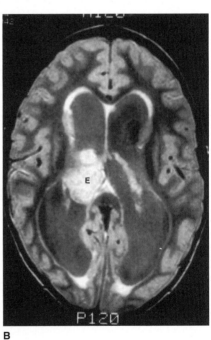

**FIGURE 14-5**    (A) Midsagittal postcontrast T1-weighted MR image shows enhancing ependymoma in the fourth ventricle. The tumor extrudes (*arrow*) through the foramen of Magendie. (B) Proton density image shows ependymoma (*E*) inside the right lateral ventricle. There is hydrocephalus.

## Suggested Reading

Furie DM, Provenzale JM. Supratentorial ependymomas and subependymomas: CT and MR appearance. *J Comput Assist Tomogr* 1995;19:518.

# Neuronal Cell Tumors

## KEY FACTS

- Gangliogliomas account for less than 1% of all intracranial tumors among adults and approximately 4% of all intracranial tumors among children.

- About 80% occur among persons younger than 30 years, and there is a slight male predominance.

- The most common locations include the temporal and parietal lobes and cerebellum.

- Calcifications are seen in 30% of instances; cysts are present in 30% to 50% of instances, and surrounding edema is uncommon.

- Ganglioglioma may cause scalloping of the inner table of the skull and may be solid and indistinguishable from more common brain tumors (especially low-grade astrocytoma).

- Chronic seizures are the most common symptom.

- Long-term survival is common.

- Dysembryoplastic neuroepithelial tumors (DNET) are rare, occur mostly among children, result in seizures, affect the cortex, are accompanied by cortical dysplasia, and are generally located in the cortex, have no mass effect, and do not show contrast enhancement.

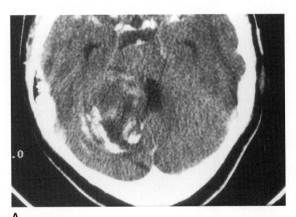 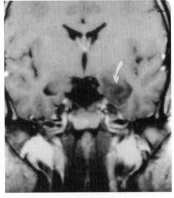

**A**    **B**

**FIGURE 14-6**    **(A)** Axial postcontrast CT scan shows mildly enhancing and calcified ganglioglioma in the right cerebellum. **(B)** Coronal postcontrast T1-weighted MR image shows nonenhancing ganglioglioma in the mesial left temporal lobe (*arrow*).

## Suggested Reading

Castillo M, Davis PC, Takei Y, Hoffman JC. Intracranial gangliogliomas: MR, CT, and clinical findings in 18 patients. *AJNR Am J Neuroradiol* 1990;11:109.

# *Primary Cerebral Neuroblastoma*

### KEY FACTS

- This tumor is generally classified in the primitive neuroectodermal tumor (PNET) group, which includes medulloblastoma, retinoblastoma, pineoblastoma, ependymoblastoma, and medulloepithelioma.

- Primary cerebral neuroblastoma accounts for approximately 20% of brain tumors during the first 2 months of life.

- Overall, this lesion constitutes less than 1% of all intracranial tumors.

- The most common locations are the frontal and parietal lobes.

- Imaging studies generally reveal large masses (> 7 cm diameter) with calcifications (75%), cysts, hemorrhage (75%), edema, and necrosis.

- The 5-year survival rate is less than 30%, and spread of tumor in the subarachnoid space is common.

- This tumor may not be distinguishable at imaging and conventional histologic examination from the more malignant and very rare atypical rhabdoid teratoid tumors.

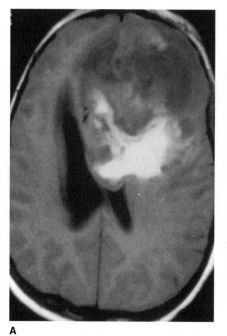 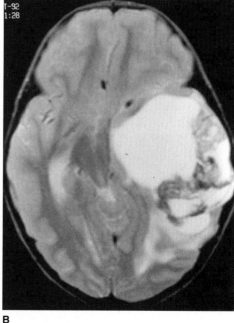

A                                              B

**FIGURE 14-7**   (A) Axial postcontrast T1-weighted MR image shows larger heterogenous and partially enhancing mass in the left frontal lobe with significant mass effect and hydrocephalus. (B) Axial T2-weighted image shows large heterogenous tumor in the left temporal lobe.

## Suggested Reading
Davis PC, Wichman RD, Takei Y, Hoffman JC. Primary cerebral neuroblastoma: CT and MR findings in 12 cases. *AJNR Am J Neuroradiol* 1990;11:115.

# *Metastases*

### KEY FACTS

- 25% of all patients with cancer will have metastases to the brain.

- The most common primary tumors among adults to cause bone or epidural metastases are breast, prostate, lung, and kidney (always include multiple myeloma in the differential diagnosis); among children, consider neuroblastoma and Langerhans cell histiocytosis.

- The most common primary tumors among adults to cause dural or leptomeningeal metastases are breast, small-cell carcinoma, and melanoma (always include lymphoma and leukemia in the differential diagnosis); for children, consider PNETs.

- The most common tumors among adults to cause parenchymal metastases (10% to 35% of all brain tumors among adults) are lung, breast, melanoma, kidney, and gastrointestinal tract tumors.

- Unknown primary lesions account for 10% to 15% of instances of brain metastases.

- Most parenchymal metastases occur at gray-white junctions, 80% are supratentorial, and 60% to 80% are multiple.

- The average survival for patients with brain metastases is 3 to 12 months.

- Metastases with increased T1 signal intensity before contrast administration include melanoma, kidney, lung, choriocarcinoma, and colon cancer (due to mucin).

- A single-dose contrast MR study with magnetization transfer is probably as sensitive for detection of metastases as a double-dose study.

*(continued)*

## *Metastases (Continued)*

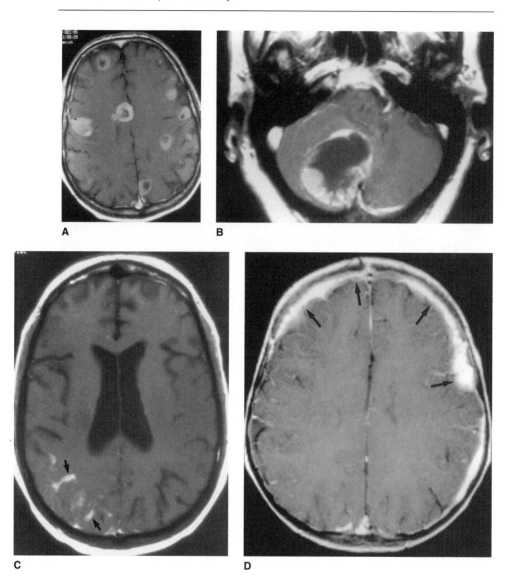

**FIGURE 14-8** **(A)** Axial postcontrast T1-weighted MR image shows multiple enhancing metastases (breast primary) at the gray-white junctions. **(B)** Axial postcontrast T1-weighted MR image of a different patient shows single necrotic metastasis from squamous cell carcinoma of the lung. **(C)** Postcontrast axial T1-weighted MR image shows leptomeningeal metastases (*arrows*) from melanoma. **(D)** Postcontrast axial T1-weighted MR image shows dural metastasis (*arrows*) from neuroblastoma in a child.

## Suggested Reading

Sze G, Shin J, Krol G, et al. Intraparenchymal brain metastases: MR imaging versus contrast-enhanced CT. *Radiology* 1988;168:187.

# Lymphoma

KEY FACTS

- Secondary lymphoma most commonly presents as leptomeningeal spread; primary lymphoma (generally non-Hodgkin's and B-cell type) presents as parenchymal masses.

- Lymphomas account for less than 1% of all primary brain tumors among adults older than 60 years but occur among 6% of persons with acquired immunodeficiency syndrome (AIDS).

- In primary lymphoma, 8% to 44% of lesions are multiple.

- Among immunocompetent patients, primary lymphoma presents as a deep gray- or white-matter lesion (most common) that is slightly hyperdense at noncontrast CT, has little mass effect or edema, and shows prominent enhancement.

- In patients with AIDS, primary lymphoma may present as single or multiple ring-enhancing lesions with edema (indistinguishable from toxoplasmosis, although lymphoma tends to abut ependymal surfaces).

- Lymphoma captures thallium-201 whereas infectious processes do not.

- Secondary lymphoma may present as dural, pial, or ependymal thickening (which may be nodular) or as a dura-based mass.

- Although lymphoma is highly radiosensitive, the median survival period is only 12 months because of a high rate of recurrence.

*(continued)*

## *Lymphoma* *(Continued)*

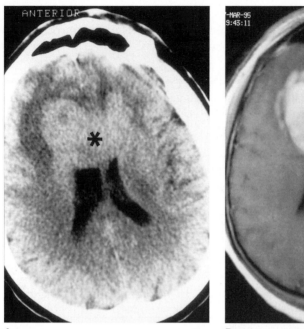

A

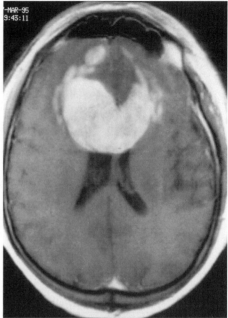

B

**FIGURE 14-9**

**(A)** Axial noncontrast CT scan shows slightly hyperdense lymphoma (*) in the genu of the corpus callosum. **(B)** T1-weighted MR image of the same patient shows the lesion to enhance homogeneously. This patient did not have AIDS. **(C)** Coronal postcontrast T1-weighted MR image of a patient with AIDS shows two nonspecific masses that proved to be lymphoma.

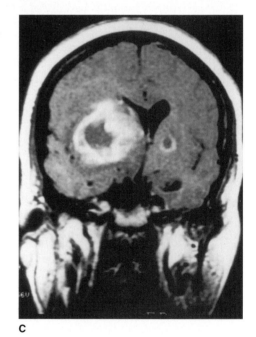

C

### Suggested Reading

Koeller KK, Smirniotopoulos JG, Jones RV. Primary central nervous system lymphoma: radiologic-pathologic correlation. *Radiographics* 1997;17:1497.

# INFRATENTORIAL TUMORS

## *Pilocytic Astrocytoma*

### KEY FACTS

- Astrocytoma is the most common cerebellar tumor among children after medulloblastoma; most of these tumors have a pilocytic pattern.

- In the general population, pilocytic astrocytoma accounts for 5% to 10% of all gliomas and for 30% of all pediatric brain tumors.

- Most of these tumors arise in the vermis or hemispheres, third ventricular region, or optic chiasm, especially among patients with neurofibromatosis type 1 (NF-1); they are rare in the cerebral hemispheres.

- Despite an overall 70% survival rate at 20 years and almost 100% complete cure after total resection, 20% to 30% of these tumors are aggressive and recur rapidly or show metastases (especially subarachnoid).

- Pilocytic astrocytoma classically appears as a well-demarcated cyst (50% to 80%) with mural nodules that enhance; absence of edema and calcification are present in 10% of instances, but occasionally pilocytic astrocytoma is a solid, enhancing tumor indistinguishable from other primary brain tumors.

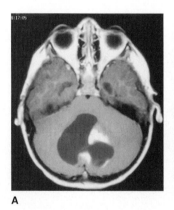 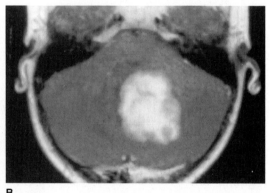

**A**                 **B**

**FIGURE 14-10**    **(A)** Axial postcontrast T1-weighted MR image shows mostly cystic pilocytic astrocytoma with several peripheral enhancing tumor nodules. **(B)** In a different case, postcontrast T1-weighted MR image shows a solid and enhancing pilocytic astrocytoma in the cerebellum.

### Suggested Reading

Strong JA, Hatten HP, Brown MT, et al. Pilocytic astrocytoma: correlation between the initial imaging features and clinical aggressiveness. *Am J Roentgenol* 1993;161:369.

# *Brainstem Astrocytoma*

## KEY FACTS

- Astrocytoma of the brainstem is a relatively common lesion (25% of posterior fossa tumors).

- This tumor occurs mainly among children (boys more than girls); most instances are diagnosed in the first decade of life.

- Most brainstem gliomas are pylocytic (55%), but they can be fibrillary (most common), anaplastic, or glioblastoma multiforme (45%).

- The lesion may be located in the pons, midbrain (with thalamic extension), or medulla; 50% involve both the pons and medulla at the time of diagnosis, and 60% of all brainstem astrocytomas have exophytic components.

- Hydrocephalus is a late complication.

- Calcifications and hemorrhage are rare.

- Enhancement is variable and may be diffuse, nodular, or ring-like.

- This tumor should be differentiated from viral pontomesencephalitis in the treatment of children.

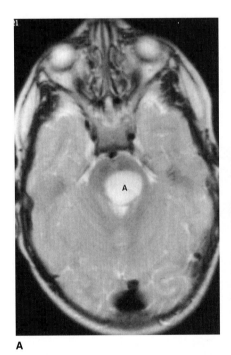

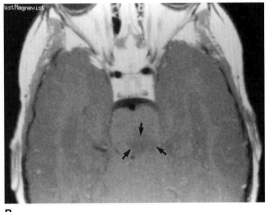

A                                        B

**FIGURE 14-11**    (A) Axial T2-weighted MR image shows high signal intensity in this well-defined astrocytoma (*A*) of the pons. (B) In the same patient, the tumor (*arrows*) does not enhance after administration of contrast medium.

## Suggested Reading

Kane AG, Robles HA, Smirniotopoulos JG, Heironimus JD, Fish MH. Radiologic-pathologic correlation: diffuse pontine astrocytoma. *Am J Neuroradiol* 1993;14:941.

# Medulloblastoma

## KEY FACTS

- Medulloblastomas account for approximately 30% of all posterior fossa tumors among children (for practical reasons, it can be considered the most common cerebellar tumor among children).

- Most of these tumors (>50%) are found in first 5 years of life; a second peak occurs during the third decade of life and accounts for <30% of all medulloblastomas.

- Most common locations are, among children, the cerebellar vermis (75%) and, among adults, the cerebellar hemispheres.

- The typical CT appearance (<30%) includes midline tumor, hyperdense before administration of contrast medium, no calcium, homogeneous enhancement, hydrocephalus; occasionally these tumors show cysts, calcifications, or absence of enhancement.

- The 5-year survival rate is 50% with combination chemoradiation therapy.

- About 50% of patients have diffuse subarachnoid metastases; therefore, MR imaging of the spine with contrast enhancement is recommended for all patients. Imaging should be performed before surgical intervention, because some postoperative changes, especially irritation from blood, may become enhanced and be indistinguishable from metastases.

- The tumor may be a part of the basal cell nevus (Gorlin's) syndrome or ataxia telengiectasia.

*(continued)*

## *Medulloblastoma (Continued)*

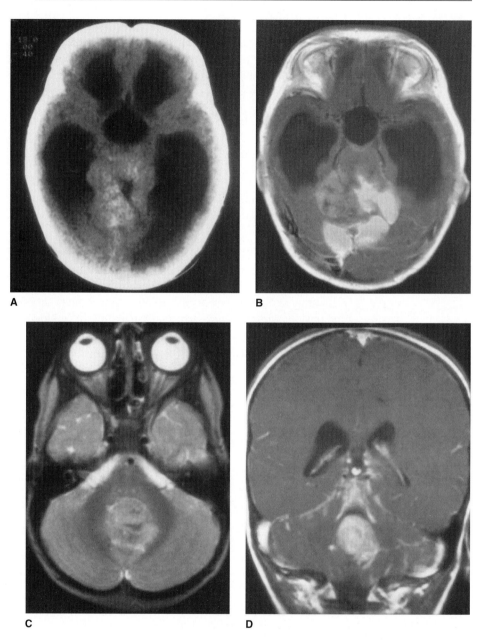

**FIGURE 14-12**    **(A)** Axial noncontrast CT scan shows hyperdense medulloblastoma in the cerebellar midline. There is marked hydrocephalus. **(B)** Postcontrast T1-weighted MR image of the same patient shows heterogeneous enhancement of the tumor. **(C)** Axial T2-weighted MR image of a different patient shows a medulloblastoma to be slightly hypointense. **(D)** Coronal T1-weighted MR image of the same patient shows homogeneous enhancement of the tumor. Note enhancement of the subarachnoid space, which is compatible with subarachnoid neoplastic dissemination.

### Suggested Reading
Tortori-Donati P, Fondelli MP, Rossi A, et al. Medulloblastoma in children: CT and MRI findings. *Neuroradiology* 1996;38:352.

# Hemangioblastoma

## KEY FACTS

- Hemangioblastomas account for less than 2% of all intracranial tumors.

- About 10% to 20% of patients with hemangioblastoma also have Hippel-Lindau disease.

- Hemangioblastoma generally occurs during the third or fourth decade of life.

- It is the most common primary tumor of the cerebellum among patients 30 to 80 years of age.

- The most common locations are the cerebellar hemispheres (80%), vermis, medulla, and spinal cord (10% to 15% of instances).

- About 60% of these tumors appear as cystic masses with a peripheral enhancing nodule; 40% consist of a densely enhancing solid tumor (most commonly seen supratentorially).

- In the absence of Hippel-Lindau disease, the prognosis is good after total resection.

- Solid hemangioblastomas are more commonly found among patients with Hippel-Lindau disease.

- These tumors are multiple in 5% to 20% of all cases.

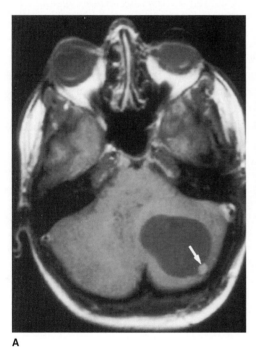 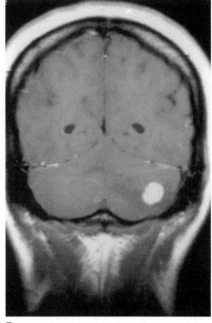

A                                B

**FIGURE 14-13**    (A) Axial postcontrast T1-weighted MR image of an adult shows a mostly cystic left cerebellar hemangioblastoma with a small nodule (*arrow*) of enhancement. (B) Postcontrast T1-weighted MR image of a different patient shows a solid and enhancing hemangioblastoma in the left cerebellum.

## Suggested Reading

Choyke PL, Glenn GM, Walther MM, Patronas NJ, Linehan WM, Zbar B. von Hippel-Lindau disease: genetic, clinical, and imaging features. *Radiology* 1995;194:629.

# 15  Infections and Inflammation

## *Meningitis (Uncomplicated)*

### KEY FACTS

- Common causative organisms of meningitis include *Escherichia coli* and group B streptococci (newborns), *Haemophilus influenzae* (children younger than 7 years), *Neisseria meningitides* (older children and adolescents), and *Streptococcus pneumoniae* (adults).
- The overall mortality (even with treatment) for meningitis is 10%.
- Viral agents ("lymphocytic" meningitis) include enteroviruses, mumps virus, Epstein-Barr virus, and arbovirus.
- Chronic meningitis is generally caused by *Mycobacterium tuberculosis* or fungi.
- The diagnosis of meningitis is a clinical one made by means of cerebrospinal fluid (CSF) analysis.
- The mechanism of spread is hematogenous from paranasal sinus or mastoid infections, otitis media, penetrating head injury, or prior surgical intervention.
- Magnetic resonance imaging is more sensitive than computed tomography in the diagnosis of meningitis and shows dural, leptomeningeal, or ependymal enhancement.

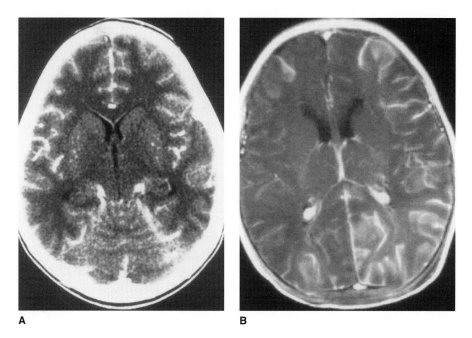

A                                    B

FIGURE  15-1      **(A)** Axial postcontrast CT scan shows diffuse pial enhancement. There
is also enhancement of the ependyma in the frontal horns of the lateral
ventricles. **(B)** Postcontrast T1-weighted MR image shows diffuse pial
enhancement (left more than right) caused by bacterial meningitis.

## Suggested Reading
Runge VM, Wells JW, Williams NM, Lee C, Timoney JF, Young AB. Detectability of early
brain meningitis with magnetic resonance imaging. *Invest Radiol* 1995;30:484.

# *Meningitis (Complicated)*

### KEY FACTS

- Meningitis with complications should be suspect if a child with meningitis has a progressively enlarging head.
- Sterile subdural effusions are more likely to be a complication of *H. influenzae* meningitis and tend to be large, bilateral, and frontoparietal.
- About 2% of subdural effusions become infected (empyema).
- Most effusions resolve spontaneously (large ones may require drainage).
- Both effusions and empyema show membrane enhancement.
- Empyema occurs among 15% of patients with meningitis; it may also be secondary to sinusitis, post surgical, or infection of an epidural hematoma.
- Empyema may be suspected if signal intensity of fluid is greater than that of CSF on T1-weighted MR images (sterile effusions should match signal intensity of CSF) and if there is marked enhancement of the rim.
- Complications of empyema include venous thrombosis, infarction, cerebritis, and abscess.

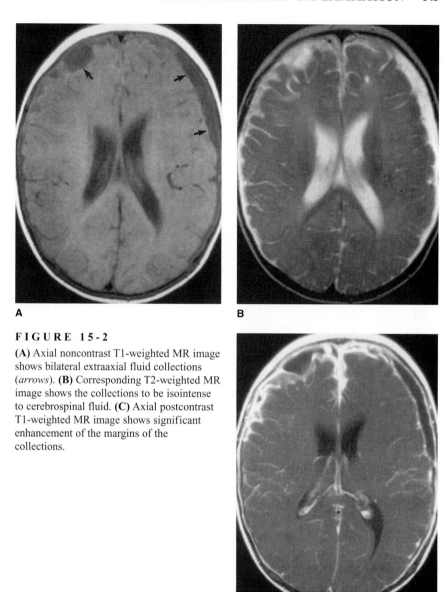

A              B

             C

**FIGURE 15-2**

(**A**) Axial noncontrast T1-weighted MR image shows bilateral extraaxial fluid collections (*arrows*). (**B**) Corresponding T2-weighted MR image shows the collections to be isointense to cerebrospinal fluid. (**C**) Axial postcontrast T1-weighted MR image shows significant enhancement of the margins of the collections.

## Suggested Reading

Castillo M. Magnetic resonance imaging of meningitis and its complications. *Top Magn Reson Imaging* 1994;6:53.

# Cerebral Abscess

## KEY FACTS

- Cerebral abscess is an uncommon entity generally seen among boys and men between the ages of 10 and 30 years (however 25% occur among children younger than 15 years).
- The mortality rate is 20%, despite treatment with antibiotics.
- Common sources include sinusitis, otitis media, meningitis (particularly among children), penetrating head injury, and hematogenous spread from a remote source (occasionally seen among patients with cyanotic cardiac disease and pulmonary arteriovenous malformations [AVMs]).
- The most common locations include the temporal, frontal, and parietal lobes.
- Approximately 90% of abscesses are bacterial in nature.
- Early cerebritis occurs during the initial 5 days; late cerebritis (with central necrosis) occurs 4 to 11 days after the abscess develops; early capsule formation (incomplete abscess) occurs in 10 to 18 days; a mature abscess is seen from day 14 to day 19; rim enhancement (in intact abscesses) may persist for as long as 8 months.
- The magnetic resonance (MR) features of cerebral abscesses include a capsule of low T2 signal intensity, a smooth capsule, greater thickness of the side of the capsule neighboring gray matter, and surrounding vasogenic edema.

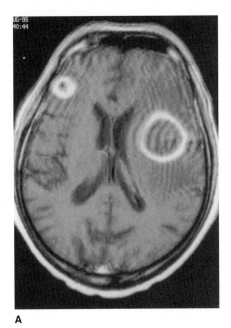 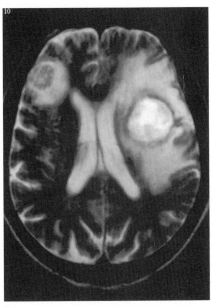

A                                    B

**FIGURE 15-3**   **(A)** Axial postcontrast T1-weighted MR image shows abscesses in the left temporal and right frontal regions. **(B)** Axial T2-weighted image of the same patient shows that the margins of the abscesses are hypointense. There is edema surrounding both lesions.

## Suggested Reading

Bluff BL, Mathews VP, Elster AD. Bacterial and viral parenchymal infections of the brain. *Top Magn Reson Imaging* 1994;6:11.

# *Viral Encephalitis*

KEY FACTS

- Herpes type I: Occurs among adults from primary infection or reactivation (dormant virus in trigeminal ganglion); accounts for more than 90% of all cases of viral encephalitis; mortality rate is 50% to 70%; produces necrotizing encephalitis in the insula and orbital surface of frontal lobes (may be bilateral); brainstem is occasionally involved; hemorrhagic transformation is common.

- Herpes type II: Results from direct inoculation during vaginal delivery (especially of premature babies); produces diffuse meningoencephalitis, which may involve the cerebellum; end result is cystic malacia and atrophy.

- Cytomegalovirus (CMV): Although rare, the most common transplacental encephalitis; most cases remain asymptomatic but may be associated with microcephaly (50% to 75%), mental retardation, deafness, seizures, intracranial calcifications (70%); affects the germinal matrix, resulting in neuronal migration anomalies; produces chorioretinitis (more common with CMV infection than with toxoplasmosis); may occur among patients with acquired immunodeficiency syndrome (AIDS).

- Rubella: Transplacental infection leading to abnormal neuronal migration and reduction of glial cells; infection in first trimester causes severe damage, including microcephaly, deafness, cataracts, glaucoma, chorioretinitis, and meningoencephalitis, which may be transient.

*(continued)*

# *Viral Encephalitis* *(Continued)*

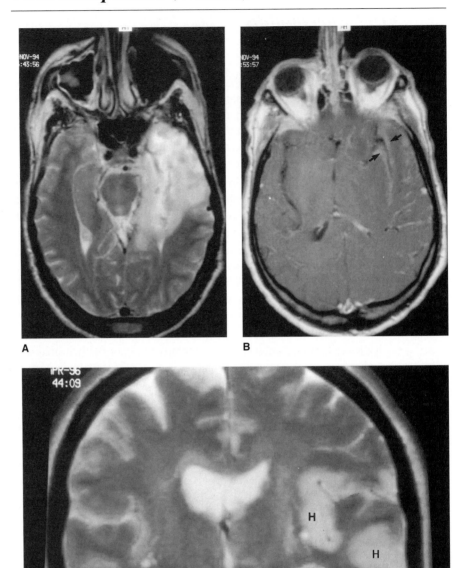

**FIGURE 15-4**  (A) Axial T2-weighted MR image shows high signal intensity in the left temporal lobe. (B) Corresponding postcontrast T1-weighted image shows some enhancement of the insular and opercular cortex (*arrows*). (C) Coronal T2-weighted image of a different patient shows increased signal intensity and thickening (*H*) in the cortex of both temporal lobes (left more than right).

## Suggested Reading

Shaw DWW, Cohen WA. Viral infections of the CNS in children: imaging features. *Am J Roentgenol* 1993;160:125.

# Human Immunodeficiency Virus Infection

## KEY FACTS

- Among children maternal transmission accounts for most cases; 2% of all patients with AIDS are children; most children die during the first year of life; and the brain shows basal ganglia calcifications, atrophy, and microcephaly.

- Among adults, human immunodeficiency virus (HIV) infection produces subacute encephalitis characterized by demyelination, gliosis, and multinucleated giant cells; it constitutes the initial presentation for 10% of patients with AIDS and eventually develops in as many as 60% of them, leading to the AIDS dementia complex.

- In adults, MRI shows confluent, ill-defined areas of high signal intensity on T2-weighted images, especially in the white matter of the frontal and parietal lobes. These lesions do not become enhanced, and there is diffuse atrophy. HIV infection occasionally results in aseptic meningitis and produces meningeal enhancement.

- The abnormal signal intensity in the white matter of adults may improve or even resolve after treatment with protease inhibitors.

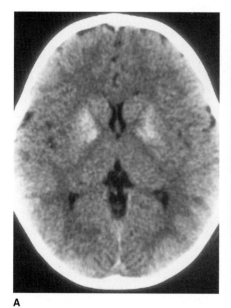
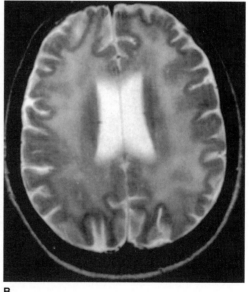

**A**        **B**

**FIGURE 15-5**    **(A)** Axial CT scan of a 2-month old HIV-positive baby shows calcification in the lentiform nuclei. **(B)** T2-weighted MR image of a different patient, who had marked AIDS-related dementia, shows abnormal hyperintensity throughout the white matter of both hemispheres. There is atrophy.

## Suggested Reading

Post MJD, Berger JR, Duncan R, Quencer RM, Pall L, Winfield D. Asymptomatic and neu-rologically symptomatic HIV-seropositive subjects: results of long-term MR imaging and clinical follow-up. *Radiology* 1993;188:727.

# Progressive Multifocal Leukoencephalopathy

### KEY FACTS

- Progressive multifocal leukoencephalopathy (PML) is usually caused by reactivation of the papovavirus and occurs among 1% to 4% of patients with AIDS; other patients at risk are those with organ transplants, Hodgkin's lymphoma, chronic lymphocytic leukemia, congenital immunodeficiency, lupus erythematosus, sarcoidosis, and steroid treatment.

- PML destroys oligodendrocytes, leading to demyelination.

- Imaging studies show peripheral white-matter abnormalities (usually occipitoparietal and less likely frontal), which may be symmetric, have little or no mass effect, and show no enhancement.

- As many as 50% of patients may have involvement of gray-matter structures (especially basal ganglia and thalamus).

- Some lesions may improve after treatment.

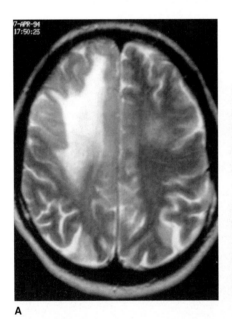
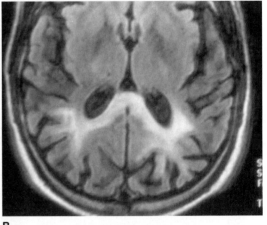

**A**          **B**

FIGURE 15-6    (A) Axial T2-weighted MR image shows increased signal intensity in the white matter of the right frontal lobe. The lesions did not enhance after contrast administration. (B) Axial FLAIR MR image (different patient) shows abnormal increased signal intensity in both occipital lobes and crossing the splenium of the corpus callosum.

### Suggested Reading

Hansman Whiteman ML, Donovan Post MJ, Berger JR, et al. Progressive multifocal leukoencephalopathy in 47 HIV-seropositive patients: neuroimaging with clinical and pathologic correlation. *Radiology* 1993;187:233.

# Toxoplasmosis

KEY FACTS

- Toxoplasmosis is the most common (20% to 40%) opportunistic infection among patients with AIDS.

- Toxoplasmosis produces a focal lesion or disseminated encephalitis.

- The most common locations are the basal ganglia and gray-white junctions of the cerebral hemispheres, but the lesions may occur anywhere.

- Imaging studies show toxoplasmosis as ring-enhancing lesions (1 to 3 cm diameter) with marked surrounding edema. The lesions are almost always hypodense or hypointense before administration of contrast medium; the lesions occasionally may be hemorrhagic.

- After 2 to 4 weeks of antitoxoplasma treatment, some healing should be present at imaging (if not, consider lymphoma); by 3 to 6 weeks of treatment the lesions should resolve.

- Healed lesions show as focal areas of malacia, which may calcify.

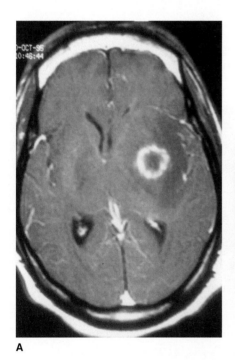

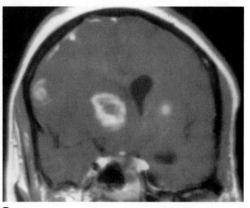

A                                B

**FIGURE 15-7**   **(A)** Axial postcontrast T1-weighted MR image shows nonspecific ring-enhancing lesion in the left lentiform nucleus with surrounding edema and mass effect. **(B)** Postcontrast coronal T1-weighted MR image of a different patient shows at least three enhancing lesions.

## Suggested Reading

Ramsey RG, Gean AD. Neuroimaging of AIDS; I: Central nervous system toxoplasmosis. *Neuroimaging Clin North Am* 1997;7:171.

# *Cryptococcus Infection*

### KEY FACTS

- Cryptococcus infection is the most common fungal infection of the central nervous system (CNS) in the general population and the third most common CNS infection among patients with AIDS after toxoplasmosis and CMV infection (2% to 5% of all patients with AIDS).

- Produces meningitis with mucoid exudate, causing a widening of subarachnoid and perivascular spaces.

- Most common imaging finding is a normal study.

- Extension along perivascular spaces may give origin to cystic basal ganglia lesions ("gelatinous pseudocysts"); 50% of these cysts become enhanced after MR contrast medium is administered.

- Involvement of choroid plexus at ventricular atrium is typical.

- Other findings include communicating hydrocephalus, miliary enhancing nodules, nodular leptomeningitis, cerebellar involvement (medial aspects), and cryptococcoma (which is indistinguishable from any other abscess).

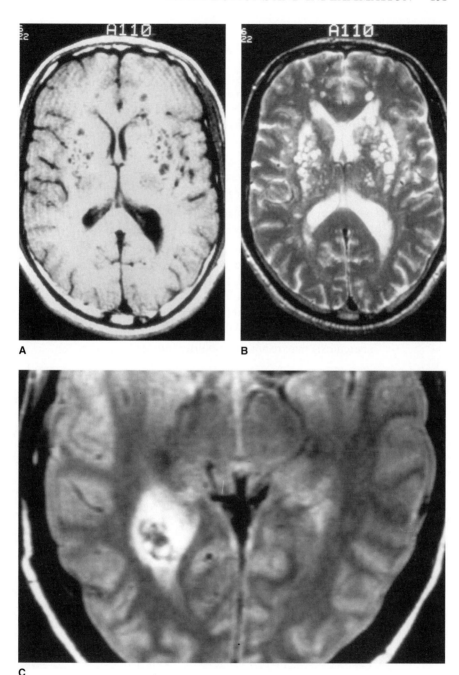

**FIGURE 15-8** (A) Axial noncontrast T1-weighted MR image shows multiple cystic lesions mostly in the basal ganglia that follow the perivascular spaces of the lenticulostriate arteries. (B) Corresponding T2-weighted image shows the lesions to be bright. The lesions did not become enhanced after administration of contrast medium. (C) Coronal proton-density MR image of a different patient shows an enlarged and bright glomus of the right choroid plexus.

## Suggested Reading

Lanzieri CF, Bangert BA, Tarr RW, Shah RS, Lewin JS, Gilkerson RC. Neuroradiology case of the day: CNS cryptococcal infection. *Am J Roentgenol* 1997;169:295.

# *Tuberculosis*

## KEY FACTS

- Tuberculous CNS infections are caused mostly by *M. tuberculosis* organisms; atypical organisms are rare except among immunodepressed patients; 30% of patients have HIV infection (particularly intravenous drug users).

- Because of hematogenous dissemination, lesions usually occur at the gray-white junctions of the cerebral hemispheres, basal ganglia, or cerebellum (especially among children).

- The most common CNS manifestations are meningitis (particularly at the basilar cisterns) and hydrocephalus; meningitis may be focal.

- Acute cerebritis may occur, which progresses to ring-enhancing lesions; lesions (tuberculomas) occur in 25% of cases and are generally small, solitary lesions (multiple lesions are seen in less than 30% of cases) surrounded by edema; calcification is detectable at CT in 1% to 6% of lesions (especially old lesions); the rims of lesions show low signal intensity on T2-weighted MR images.

- Tuberculosis may result in vasculitis and cerebral infarction.

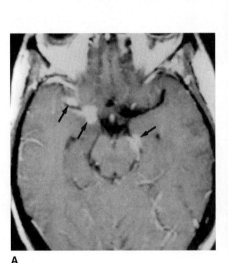 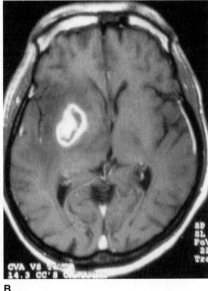

**A**                                **B**

**FIGURE 15-9**    **(A)** Axial postcontrast T1-weighted MR image shows nodular pial enhancement (*arrows*) in the left perimesencephalic and right sylvian cisterns. **(B)** Postcontrast T1-weighted MR image of a different patient shows ring-enhancing tuberculoma in the right lentiform nucleus.

## Suggested Reading

Wilson JD, Castillo M. Magnetic resonance imaging of granulomatous inflammations: Sarcoidosis and tuberculosis. *Top Magn Reson Imaging* 1994;6:32.

# *Cysticercosis*

## KEY FACTS

- Cysticercosis is the most common parasitic infestation among immunocompetent patients (its incidence is not increased among patients with AIDS).
- Almost all CNS cysticercosis involves the brain, although the spinal cord is occasionally involved.
- Hematogenous spread of larvae produces lesions at the gray-white junctions of the cerebral hemispheres.
- Intraventricular lesions are the second most common site (20% to 50%).
- Lesions in the subarachnoid space (racemose type) are the third most common site (<10%).
- Seizures and headaches are the most common presenting symptoms.
- Common imaging findings include the following:

  Vesicular stage: cyst-like lesion with mural nodule (larva with full bladder and scolex)

  Colloidal stage: cyst dies and produces inflammatory reaction (incomplete ring-enhancing lesion with edema)

  Granular stage: dead organism produces classic ring-enhancing lesion

  Nodular stage: final stage in which the lesion calcifies

- Multiple lesions occasionally are in the colloidal stage and produce encephalitis-like signs and symptoms.

*(continued)*

# Cysticercosis *(Continued)*

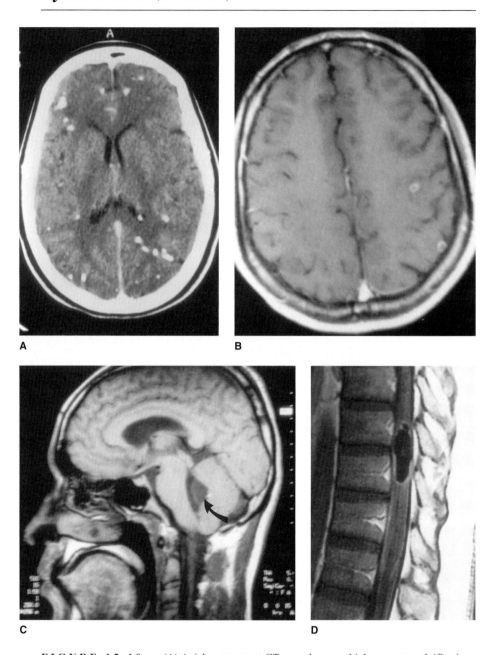

**FIGURE 15-10**     **(A)** Axial postcontrast CT scan shows multiple punctate calcifications mostly located at gray-white matter junctions. There is no edema or enhancement related to the lesions (nodular stage). **(B)** Axial postcontrast T1-weighted MR image (different patient) shows two tiny ring-enhancing lesions in the left frontal and parietal regions (granular stage). **(C)** Midsagittal T1-weighted MR image shows cysticercus cyst (*arrow*) inside the fourth ventricle. There is no hydrocephalus. **(D)** Postcontrast midsagittal T1-weighted MR image shows cysticercus cyst in the distal thoracic spinal cord. There is enhancement of the ventral and dorsal surfaces of the spinal cord.

## Suggested Reading

Creasy JL, Alarcon JJ. Magnetic resonance imaging of neurocysticercosis. *Top Magn Reson Imaging* 1994;6:59.

# *Sarcoidosis*

- Sarcoidosis occurs most commonly among African-American women 20 to 40 years of age.
- Clinical CNS involvement occurs among 5% of patients with systemic disease but is found in as many as 14% of autopsies of patients with systemic sarcoidosis.
- The most common manifestations include cranial neuropathies (II, VII, VIII), aseptic meningitis, hydrocephalus, parenchymal lesions (most spread through perivascular spaces), and occasional vasculitis.
- Infiltration of the pituitary gland, optic chiasm, and hypothalamus is typical; the spinal cord (particularly the cauda equina) may be involved.
- Cerebral lesions may have an appearance similar to that of multiple sclerosis.
- Most patients respond to steroid treatment, but CNS sarcoidosis accounts for high morbidity and mortality rates among patients with systemic sarcoidosis.
- Dural involvement may simulate meningioma.

*(continued)*

## *Sarcoidosis* *(Continued)*

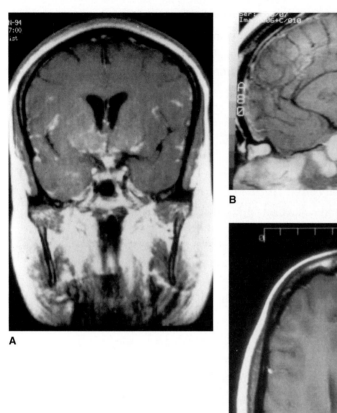

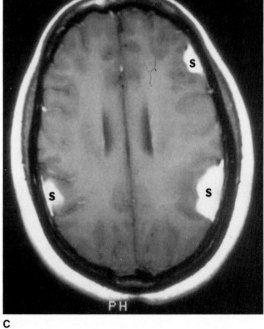

FIGURE 15-11    (A) Coronal postcontrast T1-weighted MR image shows abnormal pial enhancement. There is also abnormal enhancement along the perivascular spaces for the lenticulostriate arteries and in the pituitary stalk. (B) Midsagittal postcontrast T1-weighted MR image (different patient) shows sarcoid deposits (*s*) in the posterior interhemispheric fissure and in the sella. (C) Axial postcontrast T1-weighted MR image of a different patient shows dural and mass-like (*s*) sarcoid deposits simulating meningiomas. At angiography, these lesions were avascular.

### Suggested Reading

Lexa FJ, Grossman RI. MR of sarcoidosis in the head and spine: spectrum of manifestations and radiographic response to steroid therapy. *Am J Neuroradiol* 1994;15:973.

# *Multiple Sclerosis*

KEY FACTS

- Multiple sclerosis (MS) is the most common demyelinating disease (1:1000 individuals); it is seen more often among women (60% of patients) 20 to 40 years of age.

- MS is a clinical diagnosis in which the sensitivity of MRI (>85%) surpasses that of all noninvasive clinical tests; fluid-attenuated inversion recovery (FLAIR) images are very sensitive in the cerebral hemispheres (particularly regions close to CSF), but are less useful for lesions in the brainstem and cerebellum.

- The most common locations of lesions include periventricular white matter (>80%), corpus callosum (especially its undersurface: "callosal-septal interface," 50% to 85%), visual pathways (optic neuritis), posterior fossa (10%), and brainstem (more common among younger patients).

- Gray matter occasionally may be involved (myelinated fibers may travel through gray matter).

- Enhancement, which generally lasts 4 to 8 weeks but may persist for as long as 5 months, implies active demyelination and breakdown of the blood-brain barrier.

- Lesions occasionally may be solitary and simulate a neoplasm.

- Types: chronic relapsing (70%), chronic progressive (20% to 25%), and acute fulminant (<5%).

*(continued)*

## *Multiple Sclerosis* (Continued)

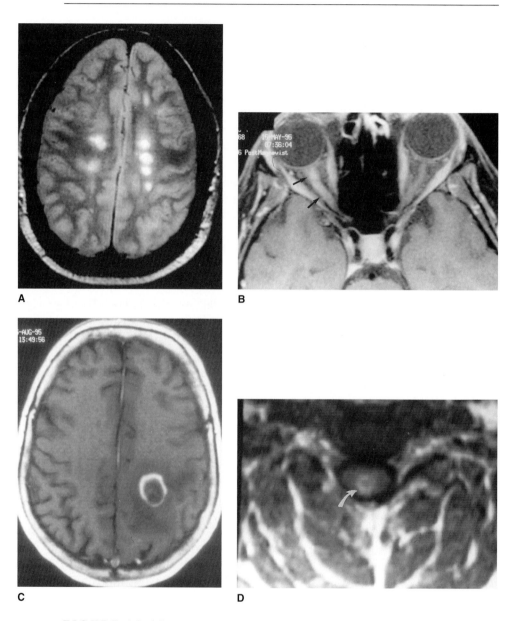

**FIGURE 15-12**

**(A)** Axial T2-weighted image shows ovoid hyperintense lesions in both centra semiovale. **(B)** Axial postcontrast fat-suppressed T1-weighted MR image of a different patient shows enhancing and thickening of the right intraorbital optic nerve (*arrows*). **(C)** Axial postcontrast T1-weighted MR image of a young man shows a ring-enhancing lesion with surrounding edema in the left frontoparietal region. **(D)** Axial postcontrast T1-weighted MR image (different patient) shows enhancement (*arrow*) in the cervical spinal cord mostly limited to the dorsal columns.

### Suggested Reading
Hashemi RH, Bradley WG, Chen DY, et al. Suspected multiple sclerosis: MR imaging with a thin-section fast FLAIR pulse sequence. *Radiology* 1995;196:505.

# *Acute Disseminated Encephalomyelitis*

## KEY FACTS

- Acute disseminated encephalomyelitis (ADEM) is an immune-mediated response that occurs 1 to 3 weeks after nonspecific viral illness or vaccination; it is a diagnosis of exclusion. This condition occurs mostly among children (5 to 10 years of age) but may affect any age group.
- The common clinical presentation includes seizures, headache, fever, myelopathy, optic neuritis, cranial neuropathy, and cerebellar (e.g., ataxia) and brainstem (e.g., lower cranial nerve palsy) symptoms.
- Lesions are characterized by inflammation and demyelination.
- MRI shows bilateral, asymmetric, well-defined hyperintensities in the white matter with no mass effect and generally no enhancement (however, gadolinium enhancement is seen among 25% of patients); involvement of the centra semiovale is typical.
- Deep gray matter (particularly in the thalami) may be present in as many as 60% of patients and may help differentiate ADEM from the initial presentation of MS.
- Acute variant with blood is termed *acute hemorrhagic encephalomyelitis* and is rare.
- From an imaging standpoint, the main differential diagnoses include MS, viral encephalitis, and vasculitis.
- The prognosis usually is good, although 10% to 20% of cases may be fatal or result in permanent neurologic sequelae.

*(continued)*

# *Acute Disseminated Encephalomyelitis (Continued)*

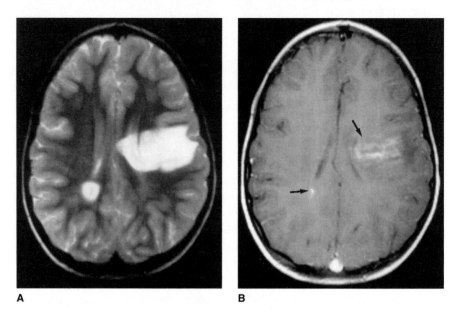

**A**                              **B**

FIGURE  15-13     **(A)** Axial T2-weighted MR image shows bright white-matter lesions. Note absence of mass effect and surrounding edema. The borders of the lesion are well defined. **(B)** Corresponding postcontrast T1-weighted image shows mild enhancement (*arrows*) in both lesions.

## Suggested Reading

Mader I, Stock KW, Ettlin T, Probst A. Acute disseminated encephalomyelitis: MR and CT features. *Am J Neuroradiol* 1996;17:104.

# 16 White Matter Disorders

## *Adrenoleukodystrophy*

KEY FACTS

- Adrenoleukodystrophy is the most important peroxisomal disorder. It is a condition in which very long-chain fatty acids are not metabolized and are elevated in the serum.
- The *neonatal type* of this disorder is rare and caused by multiple enzyme deficiencies; it involves the white matter diffusely.
- The *X-linked type* is more common and is caused by a single enzyme defect (lignoceroyl coenzyme A ligase); it occurs among boys 1 to 4 years of age, and neurologic symptoms precede adrenal insufficiency in most instances. A vegetative state or death usually occurs 2 years after the onset of symptoms.
- In 80% of instances imaging shows bilateral and symmetric demyelination in the occipitoparietal regions with an enhancing margin at the front. Auditory pathways and the splenium corpus callosum may be involved.
- Variations of this disorder (which occur among as many as 25% of patients) are known to exist and predominantly affect the thoracic spinal cord and peripheral nerves (e.g., adrenomyeloneuropathy).
- Early in the disorder only the corticospinal tracts or the lateral lemnisci may be affected.

*(continued)*

## *Adrenoleukodystrophy (Continued)*

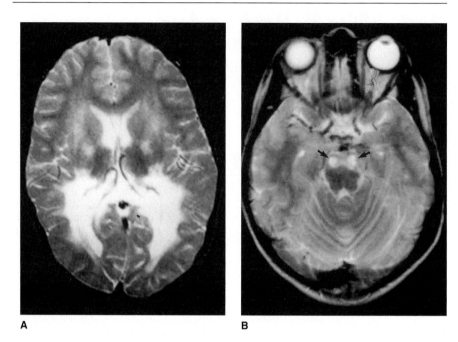

A                                                    B

**FIGURE 16-1**   **(A)** Axial T2-weighted MR image shows abnormal increased signal intensity in the occipital lobes, splenium of the corpus callosum, and genu of the internal capsules. **(B)** The only abnormality on this axial T2-weighted MR image of a child with early adrenoleukodystrophy is increased signal intensity in the corticospinal tracts (*arrows*) as they course in the midbrain.

### Suggested Reading

Engelbrecht V, Rassek M, Gartner J, Kahn T, Modder U. The value of new MRI techniques in adrenoleukodystrophy. *Pediatr Radiol* 1997;27:207.

# *Metachromatic Leukodystrophy*

## KEY FACTS

- Metachromatic leukodystrophy is a lysosomal disorder characterized by a deficiency of arylsulfatase A, which results in accumulation of sulfatides (they are excreted in urine and can be quantified) and are toxic to white matter.

- This is the most common inherited leukodystrophy (1:100,000 newborns).

- Among most patients this disorder presents itself between 1 and 2 years of age, but juvenile and adult forms also exist; this is the most common type of adult-onset leukodystrophy.

- Imaging studies show diffuse white matter disease; magnetic resonance imaging shows sparing of subcortical U fibers and areas of increased signal intensity in the cerebellum.

- End-stage disease is indistinguishable from other leukodystrophies at imaging studies.

- Death occurs 1 to 4 years after the onset of symptoms.

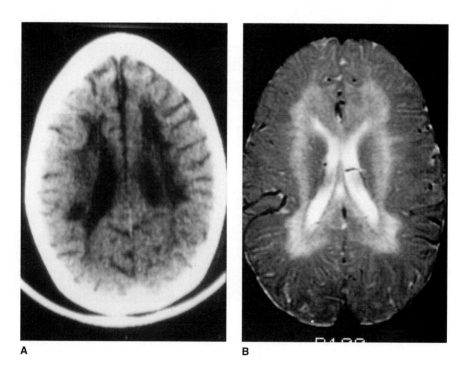

A                                    B

**FIGURE 16-2**    (A) Axial CT scan shows abnormal and symmetric low density in the white matter of both centra semiovale. There is sparing of the subcortical white matter. (B) Axial T2-weighted MR image of a different patient shows abnormal and symmetric high signal intensity in the white matter of both hemispheres.

## Suggested Reading

Kim TS, Kim IO, Kim WS, et al. MR of childhood metachromatic leukodystrophy. *Am J Neuroradiol* 1997;18:733.

# Alexander's Disease

## KEY FACTS

- This is a disorder of unknown causation. It has no detectable biochemical defect and therefore requires brain biopsy for diagnosis.
- The histologic landmark is increased astrocytic eosinophilic Rosenthal fibers, which lead to increased size and weight of the brain (clinically patients have macrocephaly); however, these fibers also are found in astrocytomas and inflammatory and vascular disorders.
- Alexander's disease generally presents in infancy or adolescence.
- The adult form may simulate multiple sclerosis.
- Early on, demyelination occurs in the frontal lobes and then extends to involve the entire cerebral hemispheres; the cavum septi pellucidi and cavum vergae may be widened.
- Contrast enhancement may be present (particularly in the basal ganglia and the periventricular regions), and its importance is uncertain (it is probably related to active demyelination).
- Among children death occurs 2 to 3 years after diagnosis.

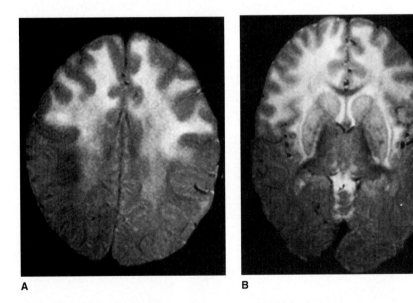

A                                    B

**FIGURE 16-3**   (A) Axial T2-weighted MR image shows symmetric increased signal intensity predominantly in the frontal lobes. (B) T2-weighted MR image of the same patient shows high signal intensity in the frontal lobes that extends posteriorly to involve the external capsules. Note increased signal intensity of the basal ganglia reflecting the presence of abnormal white-matter fibers within them.

## Suggested Reading

Shah M, Ross JS. Infantile Alexander disease: MR appearance of a biopsy-proven case. *Am J Neuroradiol* 1990;11:1105.

# Canavan's Disease

### KEY FACTS

- Canavan's disease is an autosomal recessive disorder characterized by a deficiency of *N*-acetylaspartylase.

- The brain is enlarged and macroscopically appears spongy (hence the term *spongiform leukodystrophy*); occasionally cysts are large enough to be visualized at imaging studies.

- Demyelination involves all white matter, including subcortical U fibers during the first 6 months of life.

- Canavan's disease usually has a rapidly fatal course.

- Proton magnetic resonance spectroscopy shows a large N-acetyl aspartate (NAA) peak.

- MR appearance is very similar to that of Pelizaeus-Merzbacher disease.

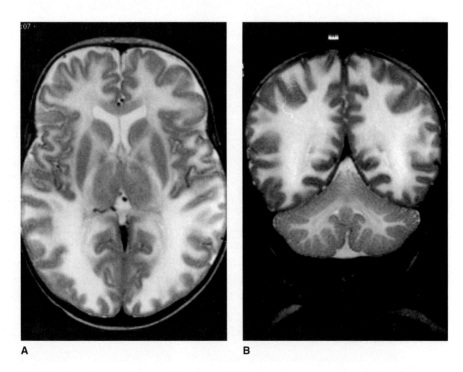

**A**                    **B**

**FIGURE  16-4**    **(A)** Axial T2-weighted MR image shows increased signal intensity involving all of the white matter. **(B)** Coronal T2-weighted MR image of the same patient shows increased signal intensity in both cerebral hemispheres and in the cerebellar white matter.

### Suggested Reading
Brismar J, Brisman G, Gascon G, Oznan P. Canavan disease: CT and MR imaging of the brain. *Am J Neuroradiol* 1990;11:805.

# *Krabbe's Disease*

## KEY FACTS

- Krabbe's disease is a lysosomal disorder characterized by a deficiency of the enzyme galactocerebroside β-galactosidase.
- The brain may be initially enlarged but later becomes small and atrophic.
- This disease is most commonly diagnosed between the third and sixth months of life; children may have dysmorphic facies and large ears.
- Noncontrast computed tomography (CT) may show increased density in the basal ganglia (particularly the thalami) and corona radiata.
- MRI usually shows nonspecific areas of hyperintensity in the white matter, especially in the periventricular regions and relatively hypointense thalami, on T2-weighted images.
- Krabbe's disease may cause hypertrophy of the optic nerves and nerve roots in the cauda equina.
- This disease is rapidly progressive and fatal; death occurs 1 to 2 years after diagnosis.

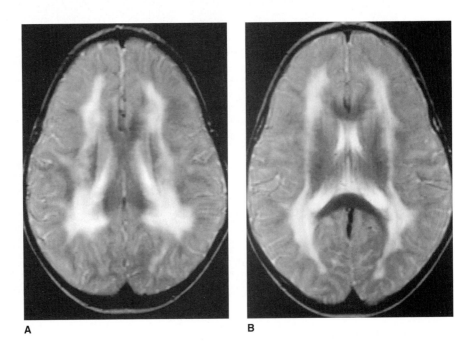

A                                                             B

**FIGURE  16-5**    (A) Axial T2-weighted MR image shows symmetric increased signal intensity in the white matter of hemispheres. (B) Axial T2-weighted MR image (inferior to A) of the same patient again shows the abnormally increased signal intensity in the white matter.

## Suggested Reading

Hittamir K, Wimberger D, Wiesbauer P, Zehetmayer M, Budka H. Early infantile form of Krabbe disease with optic hypertrophy: serial MR examinations and autopsy report. *Am J Neuroradiol* 1994;15:1454.

# *Pelizaeus-Merzbacher Disease*

## KEY FACTS

- Pelizaeus-Merzbacher disease is an X-linked recessive disorder characterized by a lack of myelin-specific lipids, resulting in impaired function of oligodendrocytes and hypomyelination.

- At pathologic examination perivascular myelin is preserved but surrounded by extensive abnormal myelin, giving a "tigroid" appearance.

- Two types exist—the *neonatal form,* which is rapidly fatal, and the *classic form,* which occurs among young men and has a protracted course.

- A lack of mature myelin on an MR image shows as diffuse high signal intensity on T2-weighted sequences. At times the abnormal signal intensity has a patchy appearance, reflecting the tigroid dysmyelination. The posterior fossa and brainstem may be normal.

- Basal ganglia may have low signal intensity on T2-weighted MR images, presumably because of increased iron deposition.

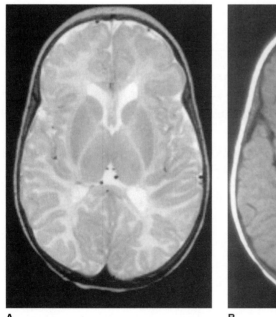 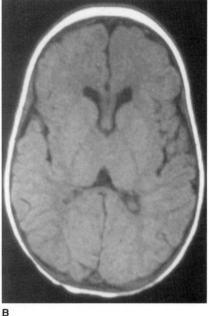

A                                                                    B

**FIGURE 16-6**   **(A)** Axial T2-weighted image of a 1-month old child shows diffusely increased signal intensity throughout the white matter. The appearance is similar to that of Canavan's disease. **(B)** Corresponding T1-weighted image shows absence of normal bright myelin. Even the posterior limbs of the internal capsules, which should be myelinated at birth, are abnormal.

## Suggested Reading

Silverstein AM, Hirsh DK, Trobe JD, Gebraski SS. MR imaging of the brain in five members of a family with Pelizaeus-Merzbacher disease. *Am J Neuroradiol* 1990;11:495.

# 17    Metabolic Disorders

## *Amino Acid Disorders*

### KEY FACTS

- In this rare group of disorders, amino acid pathways are deficient, and therefore proteolipids, which are essential for formation of myelin, are abnormal.

- *Phenylketonuria* occurs when defective phenylalanine hydroxylase produces increased amounts of phenylalanine, which inhibits a proteolipid and leads to dysmyelination. Patients are healthy at birth, and magnetic resonance imaging (MRI) shows nonspecific white-matter changes.

- *Maple syrup disease* is characterized by a failure to metabolize branched-chain amino acids. It presents in the neonatal period and is rapidly fatal. White matter and basal ganglia are involved.

- *Homocystinuria* is caused by an error in methionine metabolism that leads to abnormal collagen and elastin formation and presents as multiple arterial and venous occlusions.

- Other rare aminopathies include glutaric aciduria type I (severe dilatation of sylvian fissures), methylmalonic acidemia (symmetric involvement of globus pallidi), nonketotic hyperglycinemia, and oculocerebrorenal (Lowe) syndrome.

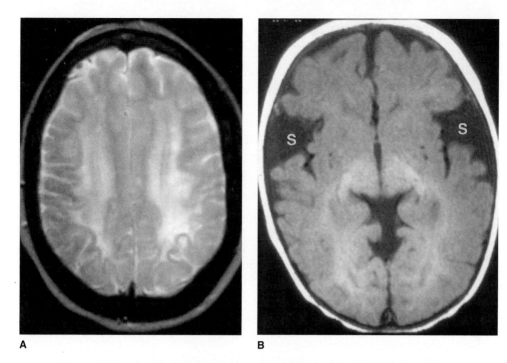

A                                                    B

**FIGURE 17-1**    **(A)** Axial T2-weighted MR image of patient with phenylketonuria shows symmetric and abnormal increased signal intensity in the white matter of both hemispheres. **(B)** T1-weighted MR image of a patient with glutaric aciduria shows small opercula and wide sylvian fissures (*S*).

## Suggested Reading

Van der Knaap MS, Ross B, Valk J. Uses of MR in inborn error of metabolism. In: Kucharczyk J, Mosely M, Barkovich AJ, eds. *Magnetic Resonance Neuro-imaging.* Boca Raton, FL: CRC Press, 1994:245.

## *Mucopolysaccharidosis*

### KEY FACTS

- Mucopolysaccharidosis is characterized by deficiencies in metabolism of heparan, dermatan, and keratan sulfate.
- The disorders include Hurler's (IH), Hunter's (II), Sanfilippo's (III A-D), Morquio's (IV A- D), Maroteaux-Lamy (VI), Scheie's (IS), and Sly syndromes.
- All types of mucopolysaccharidosis are autosomal recessive except Hunter's syndrome, which is X-linked.
- All syndromes involve the central nervous system (CNS) and the musculoskeletal system.
- Findings are usually nonspecific. They range from mild to severe white-matter abnormalities, communicating hydrocephalus, initial macrocephaly, cerebral atrophy, thick skull, thick dura, and abnormal odontoid process.
- Dilated perivascular spaces, which are radially oriented and filled with mucopolysaccharide gargoyle cells, and dolichocephaly are common in Hurler's syndrome.

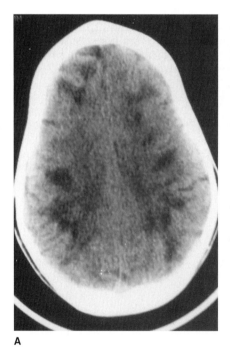 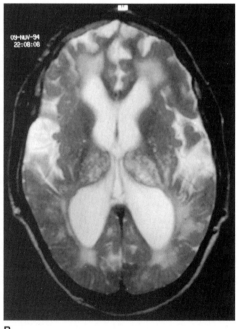

A                                  B

FIGURE 17-2    (A) Axial CT scan of a patient with Hunter syndrome shows low density of the white matter and multiple patchy areas of even lower density that are radially oriented (following the course of the perivascular spaces). (B) T2-weighted MR image of a different patient with Hunter syndrome shows atrophy, increased signal intensity in the white matter, and dilatation of perivascular spaces (particularly in the thalami).

### Suggested Reading

Walsh LE, Moran CC. The mucopolysaccharidoses: clinical and neuroradiographic features. *Neuroimaging Clin North Am* 1993;3:291.

# *Mitochondrial Disorders*

## KEY FACTS

- Abnormally functioning mitochondria lead to a defective oxidative respiratory cycle, which produces accumulation of lactic acid.

- These disorders involve the CNS and smooth-muscle tissue.

- *MELAS* is characterized by mitochondrial myopathy, encephalopathy, lactic acidosis, and strokes. It produces large cerebral infarctions that involve both white (parietooccipital) and gray (deep nuclei) matter.

- *MERRF* is characterized by myoclonic epilepsy with ragged red fibers; MRI findings are similar to those of MELAS.

- *Leigh disease* is an X-linked, subacute necrotizing encephalomyelopathy characterized by deficiencies in pyruvate dehydrogenase and cytochrome c oxidase. MRI shows preferential and symmetric involvement of deep gray-matter nuclei (basal ganglia, periaqueductal gray matter, and brainstem). In rare instances the cortex may be affected.

- Proton magnetic resonance spectroscopy may show lactate in all of these disorders.

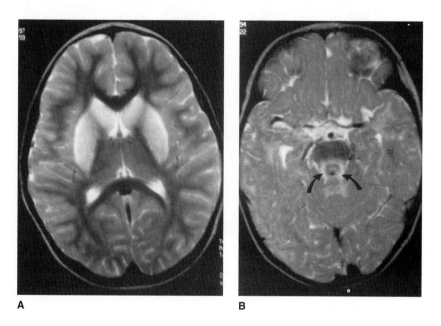

**A**                               **B**

**FIGURE 17-3** (A) Axial T2-weighted MR image of a patient with Leigh disease shows symmetric increased signal intensity in the basal ganglia. (B) Axial T2-weighted MR image of a different patient with Leigh disease shows abnormal signal intensity (*arrows*) in the dorsal midbrain.

## Suggested Reading

Barkovich AJ, Good WV, Koch TK, Berg BO. Mitochondrial disorders: analysis of their clinical and imaging characteristics. *Am J Neuroradiol* 1993;14:1119.

# *Wilson's Disease (Hepatolenticular Degeneration)*

### KEY FACTS

- Wilson's disease is an autosomal recessive disorder characterized by deficiency of ceruloplasmin, which leads to accumulation of copper in the liver, brain, corneas (Kayser-Fleischer rings and sunflower cataracts), bones, and kidneys.
- Most cases are diagnosed in late adolescence.
- The putamina, caudate nuclei, and white matter are affected, and the brain may become severely atrophic.
- Findings at imaging studies are symmetric and reflect neuronal loss, spongy degeneration, and cavitation affecting predominantly the basal ganglia (particularly the putamen) and the midbrain.

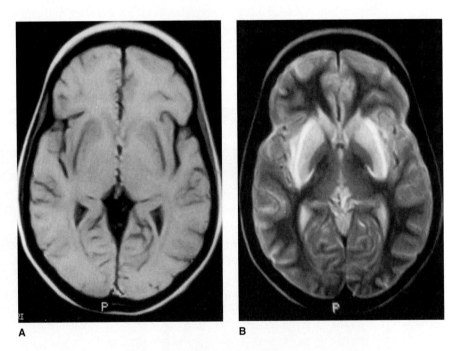

**A**  **B**

FIGURE 17-4   (A) Axial T1-weighted MR image shows low signal intensity in the putamina. (B) Corresponding T2-weighted MR image shows abnormal increased signal intensity in the basal ganglia that is more marked in the putamina.

### Suggested Reading

Albernaz VS, Castillo M, Mukherji SK. Wilson's disease: facies to remember. *Int J Neuroradiol* 1997;3:206.

# Basal Ganglia Calcifications

## KEY FACTS

- Most calcifications of basal ganglia are idiopathic and of no clinical significance.
- Idiopathic basal ganglia calcifications occur after 10 years of age and tend to be symmetric.
- Both hypoparathyroidism and hyperparathyroidism produce intracranial calcifications.
- Other causes of symmetric basal ganglia calcifications are Fahr's disease (familial idiopathic cerebral ferrocalcinosis), postinflammatory conditions, postanoxia, acquired immunodeficiency syndrome (AIDS) of newborns, and Cockayne's syndrome.

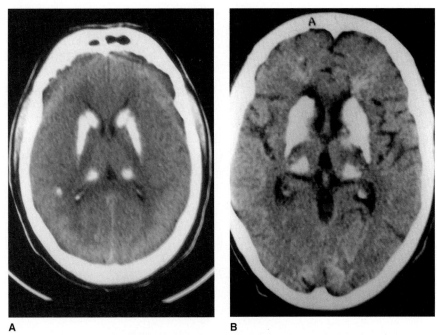

**A**                    **B**

**FIGURE 17-5** **(A)** CT scan of a patient with hypoparathyroidism shows symmetric calcifications in the basal ganglia and thalami. In addition, there is a small calcification in the right temporooccipital region. **(B)** CT scan of a patient with Fahr's disease shows symmetric calcifications in the basal ganglia and thalami.

## Suggested Reading

Ho VB, Fitz CR, Chuang SH, Geyer CA. Bilateral basal ganglia lesions: pediatric differential considerations. *Radiographics* 1993;13:269.

# 18 Degenerative and Iatrogenic Disorders

## *Hallervorden-Spatz Syndrome*

### KEY FACTS

- Hallervorden-Spatz syndrome is a rare autosomal recessive disorder with no recognizable metabolic marker.
- Clinically it is characterized by progressive dystonia, oromandibular abnormalities, mental deterioration, pyramidal signs, and retinal degeneration.
- Familial occurrence is found among 50% of patients.
- Pathologic features include vacuolization and deposition of iron in globus pallidi (group 2) and degeneration of the pars reticulata of the substantia nigra (group 1).
- Magnetic resonance imaging (MRI) shows a typical "eye of the tiger" abnormality involving the pallidum, which reflects increased iron deposition, demyelination, and reactive gliosis.

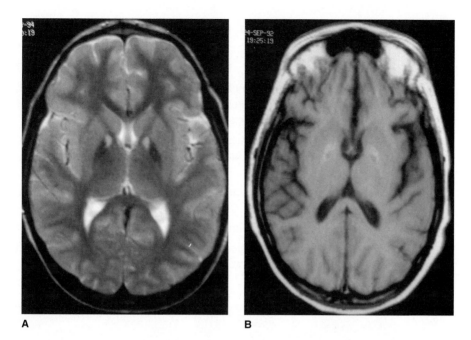

A                    B

**FIGURE 18-1**    **(A)** Axial T2-weighted MR image shows typical high signal intensity in the medial globi pallidi and low signal intensity in the lateral globi pallidi (eye of the tiger sign). **(B)** Axial T1-weighted image shows the medial globi pallidi are slightly hypointense and their lateral parts are slightly hyperintense.

## Suggested Reading
Feliciani M, Curatolo P. Early clinical and imaging (high-field MRI) diagnosis of Hallervorden-Spatz disease. *Neuroradiology* 1994;36:247.

# *Mesial Temporal (Hippocampal) Sclerosis*

### KEY FACTS

- Mesial temporal (hippocampal) sclerosis is the most common cause of medically intractable complex partial seizures. It occurs among 60% to 80% of all patients with complex partial seizures.

- The pathologic characteristics are neuronal cell loss (30% to 50% of instances) in the cornu Ammonis fields 1, 3, and 4 of the hippocampal gyrus.

- Loss of volume is more common than high signal intensity on T2-weighted MR images, which occurs in 10% to 70% of cases.

- This condition is bilateral among 10% to 15% of patients.

- 70% to 90% of patients experience resolution or improvement of seizures after temporal lobe resection.

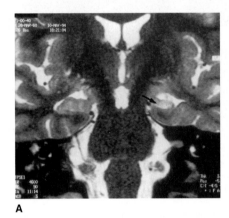 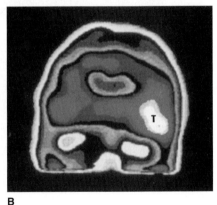

A                                              B

**FIGURE  18-2**   **(A)** Coronal T2-weighted fast spin echo (FSE) image shows small and hyperintense left hippocampus (*arrow*). There is prominence of the overlying left temporal horn, diminished volume of the white matter in the left temporal lobe, and loss of the undulations of the pes hippocampus. **(B)** Intraictal Tc-99m HMPAO single photon emission computed tomographic (SPECT) scan of the same patient shows increased tracer uptake (*T*) in the corresponding temporal lobe.

### Suggested Reading
Bronen RA, Fulbright RK, Kim JH, Spencer SS, Spencer DD. A systematic approach for interpreting MR imaging of the seizure patient. *Am J Roentgenol* 1997;169:241.

# Huntington's Disease

KEY FACTS

- Huntington's disease (Huntington's chorea) is a rare autosomal dominant (complete penetrance) disorder that occurs during the fourth and fifth decades of life.

- Symptoms include choreoathetosis, rigidity, dementia, and emotional lability.

- Imaging studies show atrophy of the caudate nuclei (particularly their heads) and of the putamen; diffuse atrophy also is present.

- In rare instances there is increased T2 signal intensity in these regions.

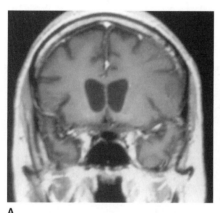 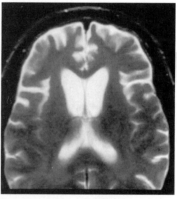

A                                    B

FIGURE 18-3    (A) Coronal T1-weighted MR image shows outward bowing of the frontal horns of the lateral ventricles secondary to atrophy of the head of the caudate nuclei. (B) Axial T2-weighted image of the same patient shows considerable atrophy of the head of the caudate nuclei with no abnormalities in signal intensity.

## Suggested Reading

Starktein SE, Brandt J, Peyser C, Flostein M, Folstein SE. Neuropsychological correlates of brain atrophy in Huntington's disease: a magnetic resonance imaging study. *Neuroradiology* 1992;34:487.

# *Amyotrophic Lateral Sclerosis*

## KEY FACTS

- Amyotrophic lateral sclerosis is the most common degenerative motor neuron disease (although rare) among persons older than 50 years.
- Clinical symptoms consist of atrophy, weakness of the hands and arms, spasticity of the legs, and diffuse hyperreflexia.
- Most patients die within 6 years of the onset of the disease.
- Histologic examination shows degeneration of neurons in the central gray matter and in the ventral gray matter horns of the spinal cord that leads to wallerian degeneration of the corticospinal tracts and of the cauda equina.
- Imaging shows atrophy of the frontal lobes, including widening of the central sulcus, increased deposition of iron (low T2 signal intensity) in the motor strip, and increased T2 signal intensity in the posterior limbs of the internal capsules.

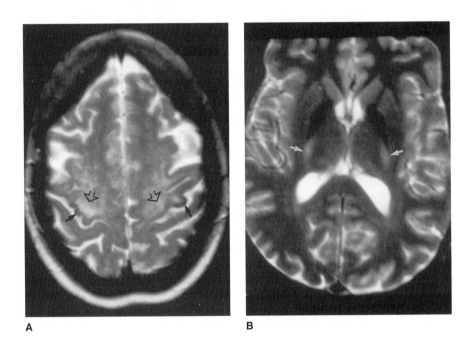

**A**                                **B**

**FIGURE 18-4**    **(A)** Axial T2-weighted MR image shows bifrontal atrophy, low signal intensity in the motor strips (*solid arrows*), and high signal intensity (*open arrows*) in the underlying white matter. **(B)** Axial T2-weighted image of the same patient shows increased signal intensity (*arrows*) in the posterior limbs of the internal capsules.

## Suggested Reading

Cheung G, Gawel MJ, Cooper PW, Farb RI, Ang LC. Amyotrophic lateral sclerosis: correlation of clinical and MR imaging findings. *Radiology* 1995;194:263.

# Neuronal Ceroid Lipofuscinosis

KEY FACTS

- Neuronal ceroid lipofuscinosis is the most common neurodegenerative storage disorder of childhood.

- Types are infantile, late infantile, juvenile, and adult.

- Symptoms include ataxia, choreoathetosis, stereotyped hand movements, hypotonia, seizures, visual disturbances, and irritability.

- Histologic examination with an electron microscope reveals abnormal storage material filling the neurons.

- Imaging findings include atrophy and increased T2 signal intensity in the white matter (no explanation exists for this last finding).

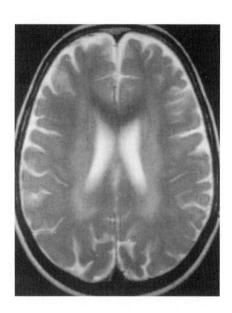

FIGURE 18-5
Axial T2-weighted MR image shows cortical atrophy and a subtle increase in signal intensity in the white matter.

## Suggested Reading

Machen BC, Williams JP, Lum GB, et al. Magnetic resonance imaging in neuronal ceroid lipofuscinosis. *J Comput Tomogr* 1987;11:160.

# Parkinson's Disease (Primary Type)

### KEY FACTS

- Parkinson's disease is common and eventually affects 2% to 3% of the population older than 50 years.
- Clinical symptoms include tremor, rigidity, akinesia, and postural imbalance.
- Histologic examination shows loss of the neurons and gliosis in the substantia nigra, particularly the pars compacta.
- Many patients have a shared form of Parkinson's and Alzheimer's diseases.
- Imaging shows atrophy and increased deposition of iron in the basal ganglia and midbrain (the distinction between the substantia nigra and the red nucleus is lost).

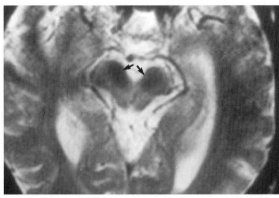

**A**

### FIGURE 18-6

(A) Axial T2-weighted MR image shows atrophy of the pars compacta of the substantia nigra (it should be seen as a thin area of relatively increased signal intensity) and increased deposition of iron (hypointensity, *arrows*) in the cerebral peduncles. (B) Axial T2-weighted MR image of a different patient shows a marked increase of iron content (hypointensity) in the globi pallidi and putamina.

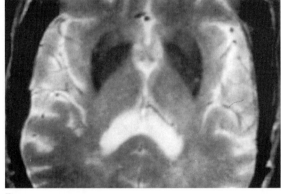

**B**

## Suggested Reading

Drayer BP. Imaging of the aging brain, II: Pathologic conditions. *Radiology* 1988;166:797.

# Alzheimer's Disease

KEY FACTS

- Alzheimer's disease is the most common degenerative brain disorder and the most common cause of dementia. It is the fourth leading cause of death in the United States and occurs more often among persons older than 50 years.
- Clinical symptoms include forgetfulness, language difficulties, conceptual loss, orientation abnormalities, and apraxia.
- The presence of neurofibrillary tangles and amyloid result in death of neurons, which leads to dementia.
- Imaging shows diffuse atrophy, marked atrophy of the hippocampi, areas of increased T2 signal intensity in the white matter (more than expected for age), increased T2 signal intensity in the cortex of the temporal lobes, and increased deposition of iron in the parietal regions.
- Proton magnetic resonance spectroscopy may show elevated levels of *myo*-inositol.

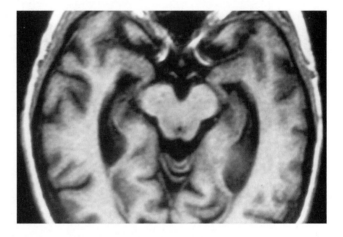

**FIGURE 18-7**    Axial T1-weighted MR image shows marked atrophy of the mesial temporal lobes.

## Suggested Reading

Miller BL, Moats RA, Shonk T, Ernst T, Wolley S, Ross BD. Alzheimer disease: depiction of increased cerebral *myo*-inositol with proton MR spectroscopy. *Radiology* 1993;187:433.

# Carbon Monoxide and Methanol Intoxication

### KEY FACTS

- Carbon monoxide intoxication results in hemorrhagic necrosis of the globi pallidi (but also affects the hippocampi and cortex) and diffuse brain swelling.

- Symptoms may be acute (headache, dizziness, alteration of consciousness, impaired vision, seizures, coma, and death) or chronic (mental deterioration, gait abnormalities, fecal incontinence, and mutism).

- Patients generally die of cardiac arrhythmia.

- Methanol intoxication results in necrosis of the retina and optic disc, cerebral edema, and necrosis of the lateral portion of the putamina.

- Clinically, methanol intoxication produces blindness, headaches, nausea, vomiting, dyspnea, and abdominal pain.

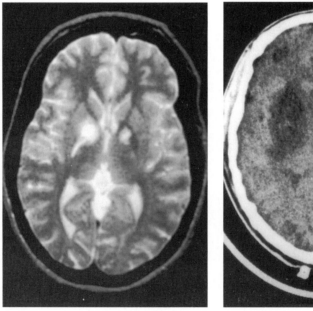 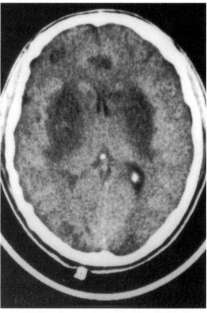

A                                                B

FIGURE 18-8    (A) Axial T2-weighted MR image after suicide attempt with carbon monoxide shows increased signal intensity in the globi pallidi (mostly in the medial parts). (B) Axial CT scan obtained immediately after ingestion of methanol shows swelling of the basal ganglia and some areas of low density in the frontal lobes.

## Suggested Reading

Gotoh M, Kuyama H, Asari S, Ohmoto T, Akiota T, Lai MY. Sequential changes in MR images of the brain in acute carbon monoxide intoxication. *Comput Med Imaging Graph* 1993;17:55.

# *Radiation Injury*

KEY FACTS

- Acute radiation injury (<3 months after irradiation) manifests during treatment and is probably related to edema. It responds to steroids, and resolves.

- Late radiation injury (1 to 10 years after irradiation, doses >50 Gy) may be associated with demyelination, focal or diffuse necrosis of the white matter, formation of cavernous angiomas, meningiomas, sarcomas, mineralizing angiopathy, and vasculitis. It is irreversible, progressive, and occasionally fatal.

- The histologic features of radiation injury are related to thickening of endothelium of small- and medium-sized vessels, which leads to cerebral infarction.

- Focal late radiation necrosis presents as seizures and is indistinguishable from residual or recurrent tumor at imaging (70% occur during the first 2 years).

- Positron emission tomography (PET) shows increased uptake of $^{18}$F-deoxyglucose by tumor but less than that of normal brain by radiation necrosis; proton MR spectroscopy shows absence of normal metabolites and presence of lactate and lipids.

- Low thallium-201 uptake at SPECT correlates with radiation necrosis rather than active tumor.

- Necrotizing leukoencephalopathy is rare and results from a combination of radiation therapy and chemotherapy (mainly with methotrexate).

*(continued)*

## *Radiation Injury (Continued)*

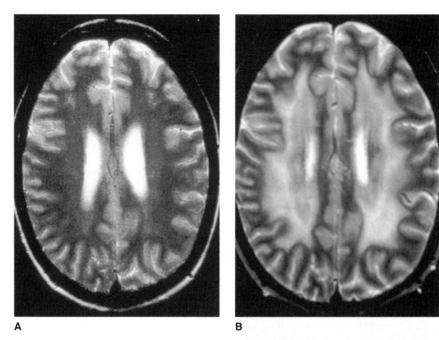

**A**                                                    **B**

**FIGURE 18-9**

(A) Axial T2-weighted MR image is normal
at the time of diagnosis of lymphoma
involving the subarachnoid space. (B) Image
of the same patient 8 months after whole-
brain, low-dose radiation shows marked and
diffuse increased signal intensity throughout
the white matter as well as some atrophy. (C)
Postcontrast CT scan of a different patient,
who received high-dose radiation therapy for
adenoid cystic carcinoma involving the left
cavernous sinus, shows an irregular ring-
enhancing lesion in the left temporal lobe that
was necrotic brain.

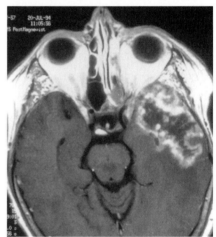

**C**

## Suggested Reading

Norris AM, Carrington BM, Slevin NJ. Late radiation change in the CNS: MR imaging following gadolinium enhancement. *Clin Radiol* 1997;52:356.

# Cyclosporine and Tacrolimus Toxicity

## KEY FACTS

- About 20% of patients receiving cyclosporine experience central nervous system (CNS) toxicity.

- Common symptoms include headache, tremor, paresthesia, somnolence, and seizures.

- Cyclosporine is bound to lipoproteins, and if the level of lipoproteins is low (<120 mg/dL), toxicity may become evident; this may explain why cyclosporine toxicity is seen more often among recipients of liver transplants.

- Cyclosporine and tacrolimus toxicity are diagnoses of exclusion (always consider an opportunistic infection) and resolve slowly when drug serum levels return to normal.

- Tacrolimus (FK-506) is a much more powerful immunosuppressant than cyclosporine and causes more marked reactions in which the brain abnormalities are similar to those seen with hypertensive encephalopathy.

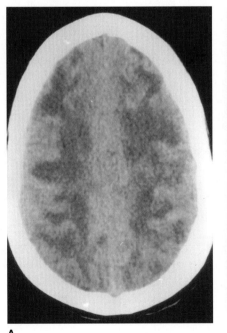 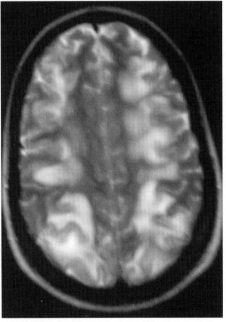

A                                    B

**FIGURE 18-10** (A) Axial CT scan of a patient with new onset of seizures shows diffuse low density in the white matter of both hemispheres. (B) Corresponding T2-weighted MR image shows increased signal intensity in these regions. This patient was receiving tacrolimus because of liver transplantation.

## Suggested Reading

Appignani BA, Bhadelia RA, Blacklow SC, Wang AK, Roland SF, Freeman RB. Neuroimaging findings in patient on immunosuppressive therapy: experience with tacrolimus toxicity. *Am J Roentgenol* 1996;166:683.

# Total Parenteral Nutrition and Liver Failure (Bright Basal Ganglia)

## KEY FACTS

- Liver failure associated with total parenteral nutrition may cause increased signal intensity in the basal ganglia on T1-weighted images while they appear normal on T2-weighted images and have no corresponding calcification on computed tomographic (CT) scans.

- This condition is believed to be related to deposition of paramagnetic cations, particularly manganese, copper, and iron.

- Normal basal ganglia calcifications are occasionally bright on T1-weighted MR images because of the presence of hydrated calcium.

- T1-weighted images with magnetization transfer normally produce a slight increase in signal intensity of the basal ganglia.

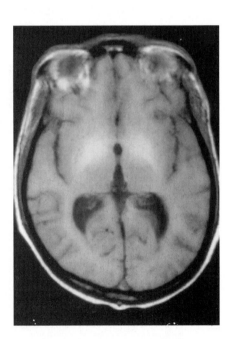

**FIGURE 18-11**
Axial T1-weighted MR image of a patient with liver failure shows increased signal intensity in the basal ganglia.

## Suggested Reading

Mirowitz SA, Westrich TJ, Hirsch JD: Hyperintense basal ganglia on T1-weighted MR images in patients receiving parenteral nutrition. *Radiology* 1991;181:117.

# Osmotic Myelinolysis

## KEY FACTS

- Osmotic myelinolysis is an acute demyelinating disorder that in most instances is believed to be secondary to rapid correction of hyponatremia (<115 mmol/L) for patients with chronic alcoholism (although this is controversial). It may rarely be seen in hypernatremic patients.

- The condition generally occurs among patients with advanced liver disease, extensive burns, sepsis, alcoholism, Hodgkin's disease, and other malignant diseases.

- The most common site is the pons (75% with central pontine myelinolysis), followed by the midbrain, thalami, basal ganglia, and white matter (10% with extrapontine myelinolysis).

- Clinical symptoms include lethargy, swallowing problems, and progressive quadriparesis.

- Osmotic myelinolysis has a high mortality rate. Imaging findings may resolve slowly.

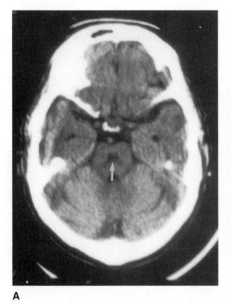
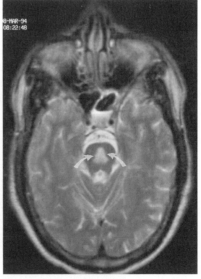

**A**    **B**

**FIGURE 18-12**    **(A)** Axial CT scan shows a triangular low-density area (*arrow*) in the lower pons. There is cerebellar atrophy in this person with alcoholism. **(B)** Axial T2-weighted MR image of a different patient shows a triangular area of hyperintensity (*arrows*) in the mid pons.

## Suggested Reading

Ho VB, Fitz CR, Yoder CC, Geyer CA. Resolving MR features in osmotic myelinolysis (central pontine and extrapontine myelinolysis). *Am J Neuroradiol* 1993;14:163.

# 19 Congenital Malformations

## *Congenital Aqueductal Stenosis*

### KEY FACTS

- Congenital aqueductal stenosis accounts for 20% of all instances of hydrocephalus. It generally presents itself in infancy but may manifest itself at any time during life.

- The spectrum of disorders includes congenital narrowing of the aqueduct (septum or membrane, forking, gliosis, or stenosis), postinflammatory changes, and tumors (especially those arising in the tectum).

- Causes deformity of tectum, which may appear thick but never bulbous (if so, consider tumor, which is almost always bright on T2-weighted images).

- May be associated with Chiari type I and II malformations.

- Endocrine dysfunction occurs among 15% to 20% of patients and is probably caused by compression of the hypothalamus-pituitary axis from enlarged third ventricular recesses.

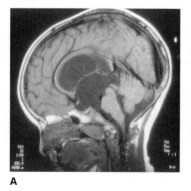 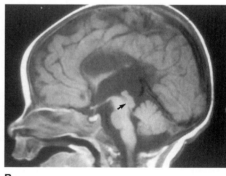

**A**                                          **B**

**FIGURE 19-1**     **(A)** Midsagittal T1-weighted MR image shows marked dilatation of the lateral and third ventricles with a normal size fourth ventricle. This appearance is presumably caused by web in the aqueduct. **(B)** Midsagittal T1-weighted MR image of a different patient shows absence of lumen in the aqueduct (*arrow*). The tectum is deformed but was of normal signal intensity on a T2-weighted sequence. The lateral and third ventricles are large, but the fourth ventricle is normal in size.

### Suggested Reading

Barkovich AJ, Newton TH. MR of aqueductal stenosis: Evidence of broad spectrum of tectal distortion. *Am J Neuroradiol* 1989;10:471.

# *Chiari Malformation Type I*

## KEY FACTS

* Chiari malformation type I occurs more often among adults (found incidentally at magnetic resonance imaging [MRI]) than children.
* It is defined as displacement of the cerebellar tonsils below (>6 mm) the foramen magnum, which in itself is relatively small; 5% to 30% of patients with this degree of displacement have symptoms; adult patients with displacement >12 mm always have symptoms.
* Displacement of tonsils of 3 to 6 mm is indeterminate; less than 3 mm is normal.
* Clinical symptoms include headache (hydrocephalus in 25% of cases), neck pain, nystagmus, lower cranial nerve palsy, basilar invagination (25%), spinal cord cysts (20% to 40%), Klippel-Feil syndrome, and atlantooccipital assimilation.
* Spinal cord cysts are more common in the cervical region.

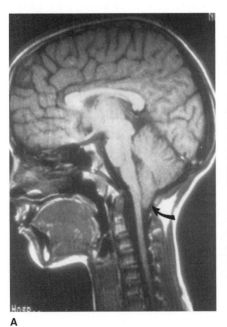
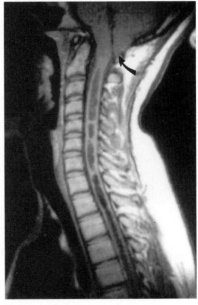

A                                        B

**FIGURE 19-2**   **(A)** Midsagittal T1-weighted MR image shows that the cerebellar tonsils (*arrow*) are displaced more than 10 mm below the level of the foramen magnum. The tonsils point down. **(B)** Midsagittal T1-weighted MR image (different patient) shows inferiorly displaced tonsils (*arrow*) and a multiseptated spinal cord cyst in the cervicothoracic region.

## Suggested Reading

Elster AD, Chen MYM. Chiari I malformations: clinical and radiologic reappraisal. *Radiology* 1992;183:347.

# Chiari Malformation Type II

### KEY FACTS

- Chiari malformation type II is a complex cranial anomaly always associated with myelomeningocele (chronic leakage of cerebrospinal fluid (CSF) in utero may lead to collapse of developing brain, producing Chiari II changes).
- Skull and dura anomalies include lacunar skull (resolves spontaneously by 6 to 12 months), scalloped petrous ridges and clivus, large foramen magnum, insufficient tentorial incisura, and hypoplastic or fenestrated falx.
- Brain anomalies include inferiorly displaced vermis into the foramen magnum, heart-shaped cerebellum displaced superiorly through insufficient tentorial incisura, beaked tectum, callosal agenesis, interdigitation of cortical sulci in superior midline, and anomalies of neuronal migration.
- About 90% of patients have hydrocephalus and colpocephaly (dilatation of atria and occipital horns of lateral ventricles).
- Spinal cord cysts are seen in as many as 90% of cases.
- Segmentation anomalies of upper cervical spine are seen in 10% of cases.

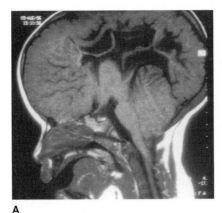

**A**

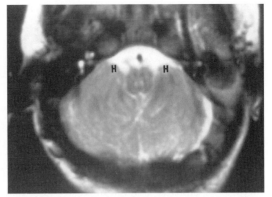

**B**

**FIGURE 19-3**

**(A)** Midsagittal T1-weighted MR image shows herniation of the cerebellar vermis below the level of the foramen magnum, smooth vermis, absent fourth ventricle, superior towering of the cerebellum, beaked tectum, large massa intermedia, and absent corpus callosum. **(B)** Axial T2-weighted MR image shows that the cerebellar hemispheres (*H*) are located anterior to the brainstem in the cerebellopontine angle cisterns presumably because of a small posterior fossa. **(C)** Axial T2-weighted MR image shows that the superior cerebellar herniation assumes a heart shape in this projection. The brainstem is small.

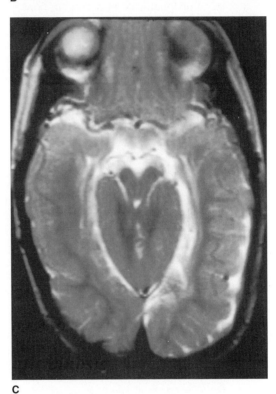

**C**

**Suggested Reading**

Ball WS, Crone KR. Chiari I malformation: from Dr. Chiari to MR imaging. *Radiology* 1995;195:602.

# *Occipital and Parietal Encephalocele*

### KEY FACTS

- Occipital and parietal encephaloceles are rare malformations that occur among 1 to 3 per 10,000 live births.
- In the United States most encephaloceles are occipital (80%) or parietal (10%). In Asia most are sincipital (frontoethmoidal). Rare types include atretic parietal, sphenoidal (associated with neurofibromatosis), and nasopharyngeal.
- Herniated brain is usually nonfunctioning because of necrosis, gliosis, fibrosis, and anomalies of neuronal migration.
- Encephalocele may contain pons, midbrain, and aberrant but important venous structures.
- Spinal cord cysts may be present.
- Chiari malformation type III is very rare and represents the combination of the intracranial features of Chiari malformation type II with a low occipital and high cervical encephalocele.
- These malformations may be associated with Dandy-Walker malformations.

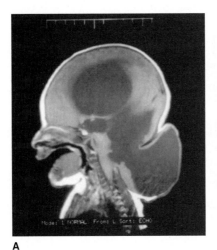 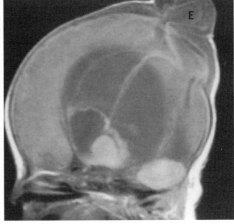

A                                         B

**FIGURE 19-4**    (A) Midsagittal T1-weighted MR image shows occipital encephalocele containing mostly cerebellum and fourth ventricle. There is hydrocephalus and agenesis of the corpus callosum. **(B)** Midline T1-weighted MR image of a different patient shows a parietal encephalocele (*E*). The intracranial contents are disorganized, and normal structures are difficult to recognize.

### Suggested Reading
Castillo M, Quencer RM, Dominguez R. Chiari III malformation: imaging features. *Am J Neuroradiol* 1992;13:107.

# Sincipital Encephalocele

## KEY FACTS

- The incidence of sincipital encephaloceles in the United States is low (1 per 20,000 to 40,000 live births); they are more common in Asia and Latin America.

- This malformation is more common among boys and always is accompanied by hypertelorism.

- Locations are nasofrontal (40% to 60%), nasoethmoidal (30%), and nasolateral.

- Most encephaloceles contain nonfunctioning gliotic brain and are accompanied by complex intracranial malformations (particularly the larger encephaloceles).

- Differential diagnosis includes nasal glioma (brain heterotopia) and nasal dermoid.

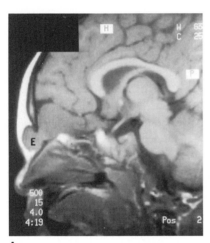 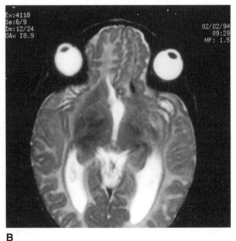

**A**                                    **B**

**FIGURE 19-5**   **(A)** Midsagittal T1-weighted MR image shows nasofrontal encephalocele (*E*). **(B)** Axial T2-weighted MR image of a different patient shows a large nasofrontal encephalocele and hypertelorism.

## Suggested Reading

Castillo M, Mukherji SK. Imaging of facial anomalies. *Curr Probl Diagn Radiol* 1996;25:169.

# Dandy-Walker Complex

### KEY FACTS

- Dandy-Walker complex represents a spectrum of malformations that vary from the megacisterna magna to the Dandy-Walker syndrome; it occurs in 1 per 25,000 live births.
- *Dandy-Walker syndrome* includes obstruction of the outlet foramina of fourth ventricle, which becomes massively dilated; large posterior fossa; high insertion of the venous torcular; hydrocephalus (80%); inferior vermian hypoplasia; agenesis of the corpus callosum (30%); neuronal migration anomalies (10%); and cephalocele (15%).
- *Dandy-Walker variant* includes mild inferior vermian hypoplasia, an enlarged vallecula that communicates with a mildly enlarged and key hole-shaped fourth ventricle, and hydrocephalus (30%).
- *Megacisterna magna* includes an intact vermis, normal fourth ventricle, occasional expansion of the posterior fossa, and scalloping of inner table occipital bone.

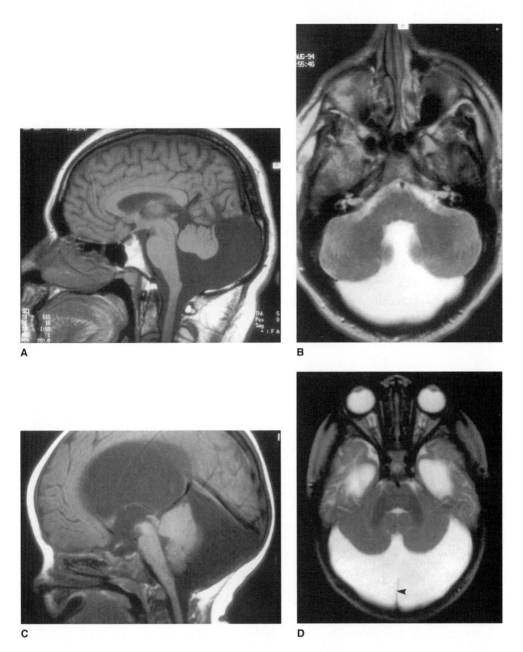

A

B

C

D

**FIGURE 19-6** (A) Midsagittal T1-weighted MR image shows absent inferior vermis and large fourth ventricle, which balloons out posteriorly. The remaining vermis is rotated rostrally. Findings are compatible with a full Dandy-Walker malformation. (B) Axial T2-weighted MR image shows large fourth ventricle extending posterior and hypoplastic cerebellar hemispheres. (C) Mild Dandy-Walker malformation (variant). Midsagittal T1-weighted MR image shows deformed vermis and a large retrocerebellar fluid collection. There is hydrocephalus. (D) Axial T2-weighted MR image of the same patient shows absence of the inferior vermis, hypoplastic cerebellum, and retrocerebellar fluid collection. The absence of mass effect and presence of falx cerebelli (*arrowhead*) indicate the presence of a large cistern, not an arachnoid cyst.

## Suggested Reading
Kollias SS, Ball WS, Prenger ED. Cystic malformations of the posterior fossa: differential diagnosis clarified through embryologic analysis. *Radiographics* 1993;13:1211.

# *Agenesis of Corpus Callosum*

### KEY FACTS

*   Normally, the corpus callosum forms from anterior to posterior (except for the rostrum, which forms last) and myelinates from posterior to anterior. Therefore isolated agenesis of the genu is very rare.

*   Complete agenesis of the corpus callosum is accompanied by absence of the cingulate gyrus and sulcus, high-riding third ventricle, dorsal interhemispheric arachnoid cyst, and colpocephaly (dilatation of atria and occipital horns of the lateral ventricles).

*   Associated anomalies are Chiari malformation type II, neuronal migration disorders, Dandy-Walker complex, holoprosencephaly, interhemispheric lipoma, migration anomalies, and azygous anterior cerebral artery.

*   Most patients have mental retardation and seizures but occasionally may be normal.

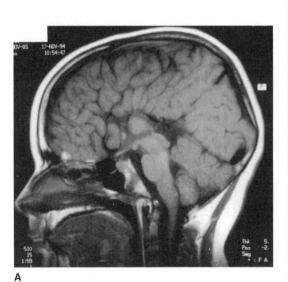
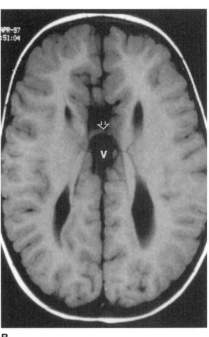

A                                                        B

FIGURE 19-7    **(A)** Midsagittal T1-weighted MR image shows absence of corpus callosum. **(B)** Axial T1-weighted MR image, same patient, shows absent corpus callosum, parallel configuration to the lateral ventricles, high-riding third ventricle (*V*), and a prominent anterior commissure (*arrow*).

### Suggested Reading

Barkovich AJ, Lyon G, Evrard P. Formation, maturation, and disorders of white matter. *Am J Neuroradiol* 1992;13:447.

# *Holoprosencephaly*

---

KEY FACTS

- Holoprosencephaly is a group of anomalies in which there may be midline cleavage of the face and failure of diverticulation of the brain.
- The incidence of this rare anomaly is 1 per 16,000 live births.
- This is the only disorder in which the anterior aspect of the corpus callosum may be absent in an isolated manner (cingulosynapsis) (see Agenesis of Corpus Callosum).
- Alobar and semilobar types have hypotelorism and facial midline clefts.
- *Alobar:* most severe type, monoventricle, absent septum pellucidum; falx cerebri and interhemispheric fissure also are absent; thalami are fused; facial anomalies are common.
- *Semilobar:* intermediate type, monoventricle but with rudimentary occipital and temporal horns; absent septum pellucidum; falx cerebri and interhemispheric fissure may be present posteriorly; thalami are fused; facial anomalies are variable.
- *Lobar:* mild type, lateral ventricles are almost normal, but frontal horns "point" inferiorly; septum pellucidum is absent; falx cerebri, interhemispheric fissure, and thalami are separated; may be indistinguishable from septooptic dysplasia.

*(continued)*

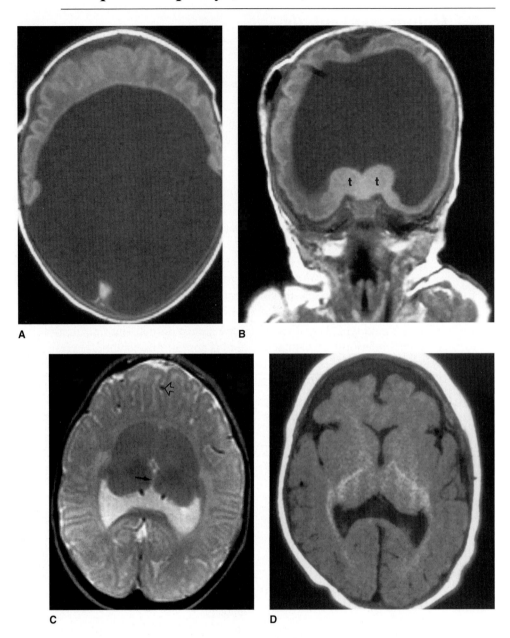

**FIGURE 19-8**  (A) Axial T1-weighted MR image of a patient with alobar holoprosencephaly shows horseshoe-shaped brain located in the anterior aspect of the cranium. There are no midline structures, and there is a large fluid collection posteriorly. (B) Coronal T1-weighted MR image of a different patient with alobar holoprosencephaly shows fused thalami (*t*) and absence of midline structures. (C) Axial T2-weighted MR image of a patient with semilobar holoprosencephaly shows fused thalami (*solid arrow*), absence of midline structures rostrally, azygous anterior cerebral artery (*open arrow*), and some differentiation of the ventricles posteriorly. (D) Axial T1-weighted MR image of a patient with lobar holoprosencephaly shows nearly normal-appearing ventricles, absent septum pellucidum, and lack of normal sulcation in the frontal lobes.

## Suggested Reading

Smith MM, Thompson JE, Naidich TP, Castillo M, Thomas D, Mukherji SK. Cebocephaly with single midline proboscis: alobar holoprosencephaly—facies to remember. *IJNR* 1996;2:251.

# *Septooptic Dysplasia*

### KEY FACTS

- Septooptic dysplasia may be considered a mild form of lobar holoprosencephaly (see Holoprosencephaly).

- Septooptic dysplasia is characterized by absence of the septum pellucidum and hypoplastic anterior optic pathways.

- This disorder is associated with maternal diabetes, quinidine ingestion, use of antiseizure medications, drug abuse, cytomegalovirus infection, and congenital brain malformations (Chiari II and aqueductal stenosis).

- About 50% of patients have a schizencephaly and classically present with seizures; these patients have a remnant of septum pellucidum and an almost normal visual apparatus; this type may not be a true form of septooptic dysplasia but rather an interruption of the visual tract by the cerebral cleft.

- About 50% of patients do not have schizencephaly and generally present with endocrine dysfunction caused by hypoplasia of the pituitary gland (posterior lobe may be translocated).

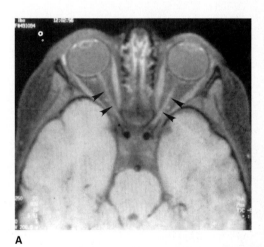 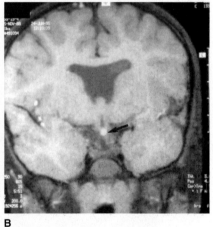

A                B

**FIGURE 19-9**   **(A)** Axial T1-weighted MR image with fat suppression shows hypoplastic optic nerves (*arrowheads*). **(B)** Coronal T1-weighted image with fat suppression of the same patient shows absence of septum pellucidum and a translocated posterior pituitary lobe (*arrow*). There is inferior pointing of the frontal horns of the lateral ventricles.

## Suggested Reading

Fitz CR. Holoprosencephaly and septo-optic dysplasia. *Neuroimaging Clin North Am* 1994;4:263.

# *Schizencephaly*

### KEY FACTS

- Schizencephaly is defined as a transcerebral cleft (extending from cortex to ventricle) lined by abnormal (generally polymicrogyric) gray matter. Sometimes an anomaly of venous drainage is present and closely associated with the dysplastic gray matter.

- Two types are *open-lip,* which contains CSF within the cleft, and *closed-lip,* in which the walls of the cleft are in apposition to each other.

- Bilateral clefts are not uncommon, and if clefts are of the open-lip type and bilateral, they may be considered a variant of hydranencephaly.

- About 50% of patients have other zones of neuronal migration anomalies.

- Septum pellucidum is absent in 90% of cases.

- Symptoms (usually seizures and hemiparesis) are proportional to the size of the clefts.

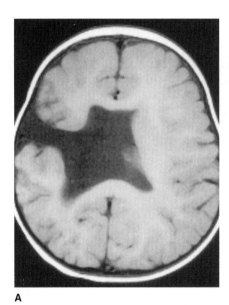 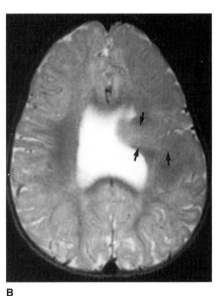

A                                          B

**FIGURE 19-10**　(A) Axial T1-weighted MR image shows open lip (filled with fluid) cleft in the right temporal region. The cleft extends from the surface of the brain to the lateral ventricle. The right hemisphere is small. The septum pellucidum is absent. (B) Axial T2-weighted MR image of a patient with closed-lip schizencephaly shows a band of gray matter (*arrows*) extending from the surfaces of the brain to the lateral ventricle. The septum pellucidum is absent.

## Suggested Reading

Barkovich AJ, Kjos BO. Schizencephaly: correlation of clinical findings with MR characteristic. *Am J Neuroradiol* 1992;13:85.

# *Agyria-Pachygyria Complex and Band Heterotopia*

### KEY FACTS

- Agyria (lissencephaly) refers to a "smooth" brain with no sulcation (the appearance of the brain is similar to that of a 17-week-old fetus).

- The complex may involve the brain totally (argyria) or partially (argyria-pachygyria complex in which some cortical sulci are present).

- Imaging reveals thickened gray matter but contains insufficient neurons ("four-layer" cortex); sylvian fissures are shallow (so-called figure-of-eight brain configuration); there is lack of sulci, and the lateral ventricles are colpocephalic (dilatation of atria and occipital horns).

- The cerebellum is only rarely involved.

- Clinically patients are hypotonic at birth but then have spasticity and seizures.

- Agyria may occur among patients with Miller Dicker syndrome, Walker Warburg syndrome, and Fukuyama's congenital muscular dystrophy.

- Laminar or band heterotopia (double cortex) is unusual. It is seen as a band of gray matter between the subcortical and periventricular gray matter.

- The X-linked variety of lissencephaly, band heterotopia, and periventricular heterotopia are inherited through a defect in chromosome 17. This type of lissencephaly occurs mostly among males, and this type of band heterotopia occurs mostly among females.

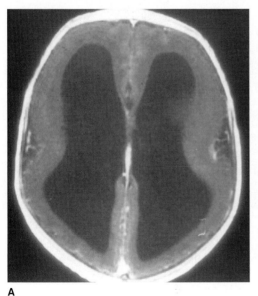 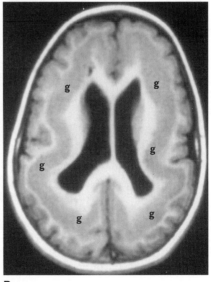

**A**   **B**

**FIGURE 19-11**   **(A)** Axial T1-weighted MR image shows complete absence of sulcation (agyria) and prominent ventricles. **(B)** Axial T1-weighted MR image of a patient with band heterotopia shows a band of gray matter (*g*) between the subcortical and periventricular white matter. The lateral ventricles are prominent, and the cortical sulci are shallow.

### Suggested Reading

Barkovich AJ, Gressens P, Evrard P. Formation, maturation, and disorders of brain cortex. *Am J Neuroradiol* 1992;13:423.

# Gray Matter Heterotopia

### KEY FACTS

- Gray matter heterotopia represents rests of neurons along migration pathways in the white matter (anywhere from ventricular walls to subcortical regions).

- The most common clinical presentation is seizures; as many as 10% of these patients have a neuronal migration disorder.

- The most common type of gray matter heterotopia is *nodular,* which is generally seen as foci of gray matter along the ependymal surface of ventricles (differential diagnosis is tuberous sclerosis).

- Multiple heterotopias may be considered a diffuse disease for which surgical management is not indicated.

- Focal cortical dysplasias of Taylor (balloon cell type) are solitary lesions identical to those seen in tuberous sclerosis (forme fruste?) and result in intractable seizures.

- Heterotopia also may be subcortical and mass-like.

- Heterotopia does not enhance.

- 5% to 25% of subsequent siblings have a neuronal migration disorder.

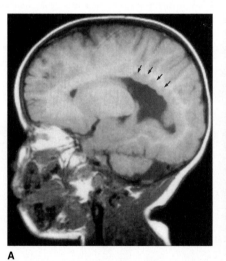 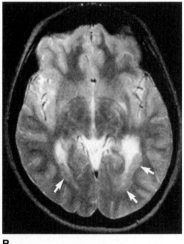

| A | B |

**FIGURE  19-12**   (A) Parasagittal T1-weighted MR image shows nodular periventricular gray matter heterotopia (*arrows*). (B) Axial T2-weighted MR image of a different patient shows bilateral periventricular gray matter heterotopia (*arrows*).

### Suggested Reading

Barkovich AJ, Cawing SH, Norman D. MR of neuronal migration anomalies. *Am J Neuroradiol* 1987;:1009.

# Cortical Dysplasia

**KEY FACTS**

- Although not a neuronal migration disorder, nonlissencephalic cortical dysplasia or polymicrogyria is probably caused by ischemia or cytomegalovirus infection that produces laminar necrosis (involving layer 5 of the cortex). As such most dysplasias occur in the distribution of the posterior branches of a middle cerebral artery.

- Gray matter may be thickened and have a lumpy surface at direct visual inspection, but at MRI it generally appears smooth and indistinguishable from argyria.

- Seizures occur among 7% to 80% of patients.

- Among some patients, MRI reveals anomalous venous drainage (persistent fetal leptomeningeal vessels) of the dysplasia or a deep cleft continuous with the sylvian fissure.

- Among 25% of the patients, MRI reveals abnormally high signal intensity of underlying white matter on T2-weighted images, probably reflecting previous ischemia.

- In rare instances, this abnormality shows calcifications on computed tomographic (CT) scans.

*(continued)*

## *Cortical Dysplasia* (Continued)

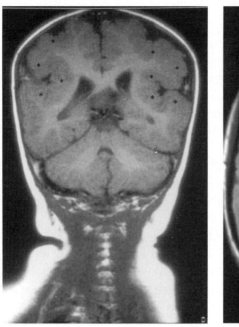
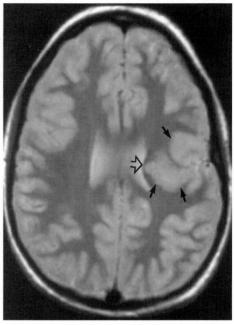

A                                    B

FIGURE 19-13     **(A)** Coronal T1-weighted MR image shows bilateral posterior perisylvian cortical dysplasia (*). **(B)** Axial T2-weighted MR image of a different patient shows left perisylvian cortical dysplasia (*arrows*). This is not schizencephaly because a thin band of white matter (*open arrow*) separates the dysplastic gray matter from the lateral ventricle.

### Suggested Reading

Barkovich AJ, Kjos BO. Nonlissencephalic cortical dysplasias: correlation of imaging findings with clinical deficits. *Am J Neuroradiol* 1992;13:95.

# Megalencephaly

### KEY FACTS

- The *generalized* type of megalencephaly is usually idiopathic but occasionally occurs with pituitary gigantism, neurofibromatosis type 1, metabolic disorders (e.g., mucopolysaccharidosis), and leukodystrophy (e.g., Alexander's disease and Canavan's disease).

- The *unilateral* type represents a hamartomatous malformation of one cerebral hemisphere. It presents with seizures, hemiplegia, and developmental delay; it may be associated with the linear sebaceous nevus syndrome, hypomelanosis of Ito, and neurofibromatosis type 1.

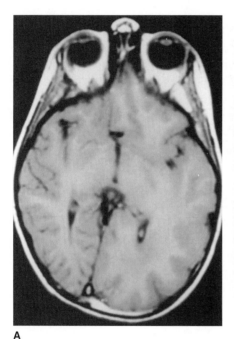 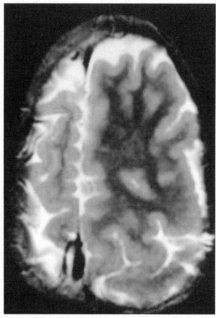

**A**                                              **B**

**FIGURE 19-14**    **(A)** Axial T1-weighted MR image shows large left hemisphere with diffusely abnormal cortex. **(B)** Axial T2-weighted MR image of the same patient shows large left hemisphere with diffusely abnormal gray matter.

### Suggested Reading

Barkovich AJ, Cawing SH. Unilateral megalencephaly: correlation of MR imaging and pathologic characteristics. *Am J Neuroradiol* 1990;11:523.

# 20 Neurocutaneous Syndromes

## Neurofibromatosis Type 1, Astrocytoma

### KEY FACTS

- Neurofibromatosis type 1 (NF-1) with astrocytoma is an autosomal dominant (chromosome 17) disorder that is ten times more common than neurofibromatosis type 2 (NF-2). Prominent cutaneous lesions, plexiform neurofibromas, and bilateral optic nerve gliomas (the hallmark of the disease) occur.

- This disorder is associated with tumors that originate from cells that form the brain, i.e., glial cells and neurons (gliomas and hamartomas).

- About 15% to 40% of patients have optic pathway gliomas. Most (>80%) of the tumors are slow growing (some even regress) and can be considered "hamartomas."

- About 10% of patients have brain gliomas that involve mainly the brainstem and tectum (producing hydrocephalus); most are low grade.

- Other intracranial abnormalities include hamartoma, dysplasia of the greater wing of the sphenoid leading to pulsatile exophthalmos, and neurofibroma arising from cranial nerves.

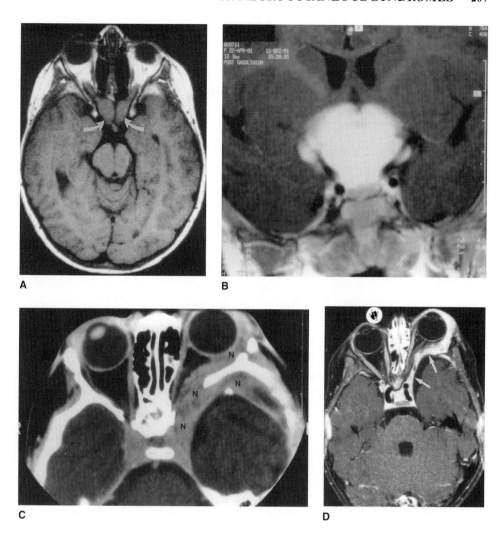

**FIGURE 20-1** (A) Axial noncontrast T1-weighted MR image shows presumed astrocytomas (*arrows*) involving the prechiasmatic optic nerves. (B) Coronal postcontrast T1-weighted MR image of a different patient shows enhancing optic chiasm astrocytoma. (C) Axial CT scan of a different patient shows dysplasia of the left greater sphenoidal wing. A plexiform neurofibroma (*N*) extends from the left cavernous sinus to the left orbit. There is proptosis. (D) Corresponding postcontrast T1-weighted MR image shows enhancement of the plexiform neurofibroma (*arrows*).

## Suggested Reading
Smirniotopoulos JG, Murphy FM. The phakomatoses. *Am J Neuroradiol* 1992;13:725.

# Neurofibromatosis Type 1, Myelin Vacuolization

### KEY FACTS

- Myelin vacuolization, previously known as hamartoma, are areas of dysplastic neurons and microcytes; found in nearly 80% of patients with NF-1.

- Myelin vacuolization occurs predominantly in the basal ganglia (at the globus pallidus they tend to be larger and may be slightly hyperintense on precontrast T1-weighted magnetic resonance [MR] images) and in the optic radiations, internal capsules, corpus callosum, brainstem, and cerebellar and cerebral peduncles.

- At magnetic resonance imaging (MRI) these lesions generally show no mass effect, do not become enhanced, and may grow slowly until the patient reaches 10 years of age, after which they usually begin to regress.

- At MRI, most areas of myelin vacuolization are isointense or hyperintense on T1-weighted images, whereas most astrocytomas are hypointense; on T2-weighted images the areas are hyperintense, reflecting their spongiform nature.

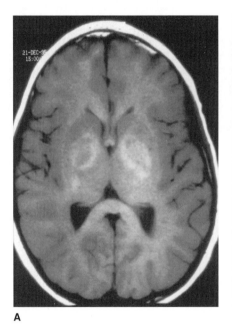 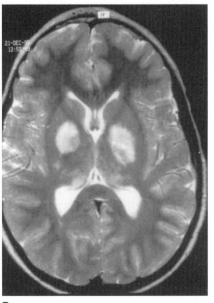

A                              B

**F I G U R E   2 0 - 2**    **(A)** Noncontrast axial T1-weighted MR image shows bright areas of myelin vacuolization in the globi pallidi. **(B)** Corresponding T2-weighted image shows the abnormalities to be hyperintense.

### Suggested Reading

DiPaolo DP, Zimmerman RA, Rorke LB, Zackai EH, Bilaniuk LT, Yachnis AT. Neurofibromatosis type 1: pathologic substrate of high-signal-intensity foci in the brain. *Radiology* 1995;195:721.

# *Spinal Abnormalities with Neurofibromatosis Types 1 and 2*

## KEY FACTS

- More than 60% of patients with NF-1 have spinal abnormalities.

- Bone changes include expansion of the neuroforamina, widening of the spinal canal, and scalloping of the posterior aspect of the vertebral bodies; these changes may be caused by neurofibromas (10% to 20% of patients with NF-1) or more commonly by dural ectasia and arachnoid cysts.

- Acute angle kyphoscoliosis is typical of NF-1 (scoliosis is more common with NF-1).

- Lateral thoracic meningocele is characteristic of NF-1 (if incidentally discovered, a search for other stigmata of NF-1 is recommended).

- Spinal cord lesions are gliomas (10% to 15% of patients with NF-1) or in rare instances hamartomas and ependymomas and schwannomas in NF-2; spinal tumors are overall more common with NF-2.

- Dural and bone changes are more common with NF-1, whereas tumors are more common in NF-2.

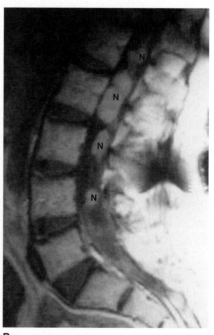

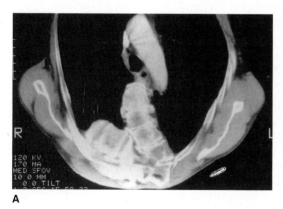

**A**

**B**

**FIGURE 20-3** (A) Axial CT scan shows acute-angle thoracic kyphoscoliosis. (B) Postcontrast midsagittal T1-weighted MR image shows multiple intradural neurofibromas (*N*) in the lumbar region.

## Suggested Reading

Mautner VF, Tatagiba M, Lindenau M, et al. Spinal tumors in patients with neurofibromatosis type 2: MR imaging study of frequency, multiplicity, and variety. *Am J Roentgenol* 1995;165:951.

# Neurofibromatosis Type 2, Schwannoma and Meningioma

## KEY FACTS

- This autosomal dominant (chromosome 22) disorder is 10 times less common than NF-1; cutaneous lesions are less common (<50%).

- This disorder generally presents itself in the third and fourth decades of life; all patients have tumors of the central nervous system.

- Bilateral vestibular nerve schwannomas are the hallmark sign; the trigeminal is the second most commonly involved cranial nerve (a tumor originating in a purely motor cranial nerve should prompt a search for NF-2).

- Brain lesions arise from the coverings of the brain, i.e., Schwann's, meningeal, and ependymal cells (schwannomas, meningiomas, and ependymomas).

- Meningiomas in patients with NF-2 are usually multiple and occur in atypical locations.

- Meningioma in a child should raise suspicion of NF-2.

- Meningiomas in patients with NF-2 present more commonly in the lateral ventricles than do sporadic meningiomas (16% versus 5%).

- The histologic features of most meningiomas among patients with NF-2 are fibroblastic subtype; therefore the lesions are of low signal intensity on T2-weighted MR images.

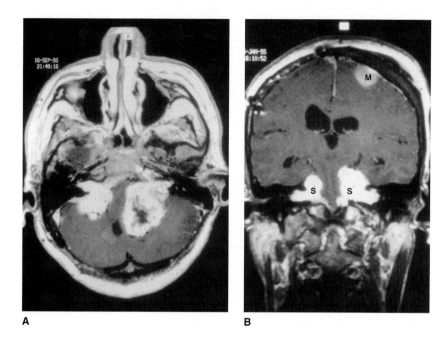

**FIGURE 20-4** **(A)** Postcontrast axial T1-weighted MR image shows bilateral, large, enhancing vestibular schwannomas. **(B)** Postcontrast coronal T1-weighted image of a different patient shows bilateral vestibular schwannomas (*S*) and a meningioma (*M*).

## Suggested Reading

Starshak RJ. Chromosome 22: a model with implications for diagnostic imaging. *Am J Roentgenol* 1996;167:315.

# *Tuberous Sclerosis, Hamartoma*

### KEY FACTS

- Tuberous sclerosis with cerebral hamartomas is an autosomal dominant disorder probably related to abnormalities in chromosomes 9 and 16. It occurs among 1 per 10,000 to 20,000 live births.

- A classic triad (<50%) includes facial angiofibromas, seizures (80% to 100% of patients), and mental retardation.

- About 95% of patients show brain hamartomas at MRI; therefore hamartomas (particularly subcortical ones) are the imaging hallmark of this disease.

- Hamartomas are composed of disordered glial tissue, heterotopic neurons, giant cells, and calcifications (which may be entirely absent, especially in early life).

- Hamartomas occur in periventricular regions or anywhere in the white matter (as many as 90% of instances); they are seen on T2-weighted MR images, are wedge-shaped, may have a slight mass effect. Ten percent enhance. Computed tomographic (CT) scans often show calcification, particularly after 10 years of age.

- The cortex overlying hamartomas is usually smooth. On T2-weighted images there is often a linear hyperintensity extending from the subcortical hamartoma to the ipsilateral ventricle.

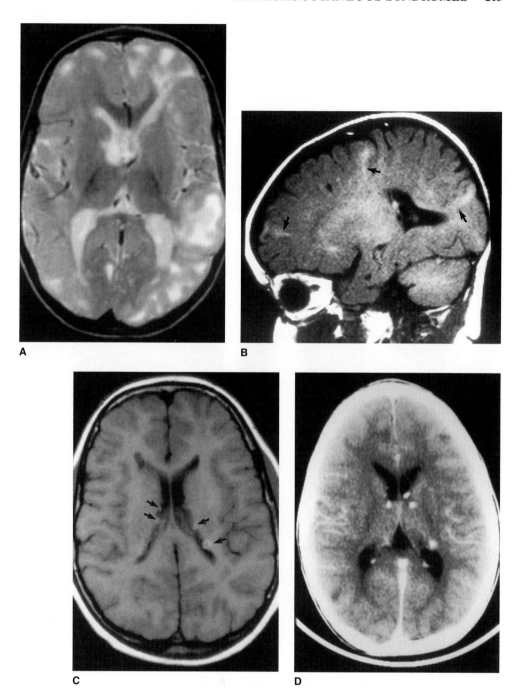

**FIGURE 20-5** **(A)** Axial T2-weighted MR image shows multiple subcortical and periventricular bright hamartomas. **(B)** Parasagittal T1-weighted MR image of a different patient shows slightly bright linear areas (*arrows*) extending from subcortical to periventricular regions. **(C)** Noncontrast axial T1-weighted MR image of a different patient shows slightly bright periventricular hamartomas (*arrows*). **(D)** CT scan of a different patient shows multiple calcified periventricular hamartomas.

## Suggested Reading

Braffman BH, Bilaniuk LT, Naidich TP, et al: MR imaging of tuberous sclerosis: pathogenesis, use of gadopentetate dimeglumine, and literature review. *Radiology* 1992;183:227.

# Tuberous Sclerosis, Subependymal Giant Cell Astrocytoma

## KEY FACTS

- Subependymal giant cell astrocytoma develops in 5% to 15% of patients with tuberous sclerosis.
- Most commonly originate from degeneration of subependymal hamartomas at the level of the foramina of Monro (slight right-sided preference) but they may occur anywhere in the brain.
- These tumors are histologically benign but may occasionally invade the brain.
- The tumor grows slowly, leading to unilateral or bilateral dilatation of the lateral ventricles; although indistinguishable from enhancing hamartomas, when small, giant cell astrocytomas show growth at sequential imaging studies.

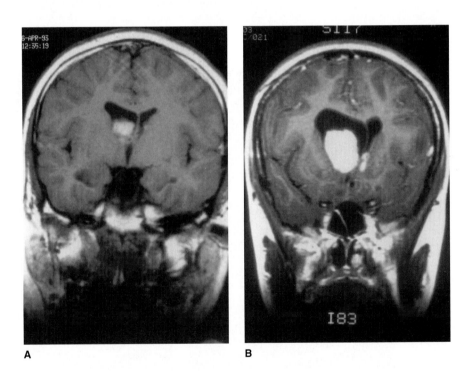

**A**                                                  **B**

**FIGURE 20-6**    (A) Coronal postcontrast T1-weighted MR image shows an enhancing giant cell astrocytoma in the region of the right foramen of Monro. The right lateral ventricle is prominent. (B) Corresponding image obtained 2 years later shows marked growth of the right-sided tumor and development of a tumor in the region of the left foramen of Monro. There is hydrocephalus and mass effect on the cortical sulci.

## Suggested Reading

Seidenwurm DJ, Barkovich AJ. Understanding tuberous sclerosis. *Radiology* 1992;183:23.

# *von Hippel-Lindau Disease*

## KEY FACTS

- Von Hippel-Lindau disease is an autosomal dominant disorder linked to a defect in chromosome 3 (defective tumor suppressor gene). It occurs among 1 in 35,000 to 40,000 live births.

- Central nervous system (CNS) lesions become symptomatic between 20 and 50 years of age.

- Hemangioblastomas (multiple ones are found among 10% of patients) are the hallmark of this disorder and are seen in as many as 50% of patients with von Hippel-Lindau disease.

- About 65% of hemangioblastomas occur in the cerebellum, 15% in the spinal cord, and 20% in the brainstem.

- Retinal angiomas are present in half of the patients and are very small. At imaging the most common eye finding is retinal detachment.

- About 20% to 40% of hemangioblastomas are solid. Most are typically cystic (60% to 80%) with a mural nodule, which tends to be subpial in location.

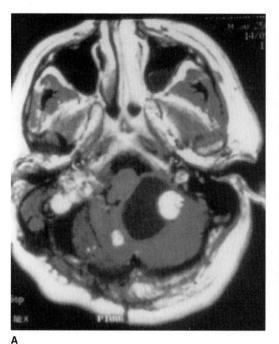 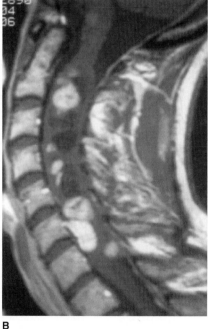

A                                              B

**FIGURE 20-7**   **(A)** Axial postcontrast T1-weighted MR image shows a left-sided cystic hemangioblastoma and multiple small solid ones in the right cerebellar hemisphere. **(B)** Midsagittal postcontrast T1-weighted MR image of a different patient shows multiple solid and cystic hemangioblastomas in the cervical spinal cord.

## Suggested Reading

Choyke PL, Glenn GM, Walther MM, Patronas NJ, Linehan WM, Zbar B. von Hippel-Lindau disease: genetic, clinical, and imaging features. *Radiology* 1995;194:629.

# Sturge-Weber Syndrome

### KEY FACTS

- Sturge-Weber syndrome is a disorder of the vascular system that involves the face, brain, and meninges.
- The pattern of inheritance is not known.
- Although patients are healthy at birth, 90% experience seizures, dementia, hemiplegia, and visual defects during their lifetimes.
- Port-wine nevi are located in the trigeminal nerve distribution (particularly the first division), and an ipsilateral occipitoparietal venous angioma is present within the leptomeninges.
- Cortical veins do not develop in the area where pial angioma is located and lead to blood stasis with secondary dystrophic calcification of underlying cortex (infarction?).
- The involved cerebral hemisphere eventually becomes atrophic.
- Brain calcifications are uncommon before 2 years of age.
- Bilateral involvement is very rare.

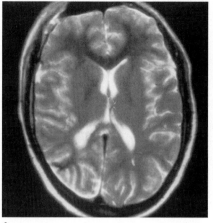

**A**

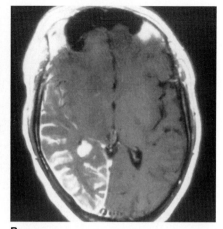

**B**

### FIGURE 20-8

**(A)** Axial T2-weighted MR image shows some atrophy and hypointensity in the right occipital lobe. **(B)** Corresponding postcontrast T1-weighted image shows extensive enhancement of the leptomeningeal angioma and a prominent glomus of the right choroid plexus, which serves for collateral venous drainage. **(C)** Axial CT scan of an adult shows parenchymal calcification in the right parietal lobe.

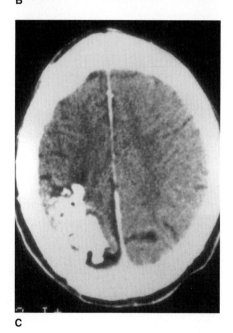

**C**

## Suggested Reading

Benedict RA, Brown DC, Ghat V, et al. Sturge-Weber syndrome: cranial MR with Gd-DTPA. *Am J Neuroradiol* 1993;14:409.

*Section B*

# *SPINE*

# 21 Degenerative Spine

## *Herniated Disc, Lumbar Spine*

### KEY FACTS

- By 18 years of age 28% of the U.S. population show degenerative changes in the spine, and after 50 years of age 85% to 95% show degenerative changes. Low signal intensity on T2-weighted MR images probably reflects loss of proteoglycans and indicates degenerative changes.
- Almost all lumbar herniated discs occur at L4-5 and L5-S1 and are central or slightly eccentric in location.
- Herniation of a disc implies a tear in the annulus fibrosus with posterior protrusion or extrusion of the nucleus pulposus, which is contained by an intact posterior longitudinal ligament (subligamentous).
- Central and slightly eccentric herniated discs affect the roots exiting at the level immediately below.
- Nearly 90% of persons with disc herniation show clinical improvement after 8 to 10 weeks of symptomatic treatment, 50% have considerable reduction in size of herniation at magnetic resonance imaging (MRI), and only 8% to 10% become worse.

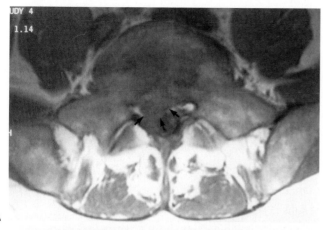

A

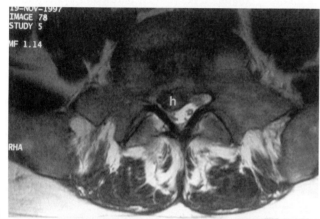

B

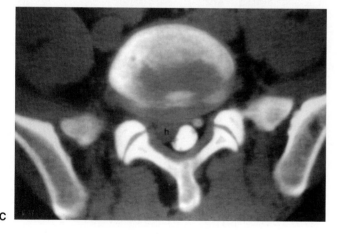

C

**FIGURE 21-1**

**(A)** Axial T1-weighted MR image shows a central and rightward disc herniation (*arrows*) at L5-S1. **(B)** Corresponding T2-weighted image shows the herniated disc (*h*). **(C)** Axial postmyelographic CT scan of a different patient shows rightward disc herniation (*h*) with compression of the right S1 nerve root.

## Suggested Reading

Bozzao A, Gallluci M, Masciocchil C, Aprile I, Barile A, Passariello R. Lumbar disk herniation: MR imaging assessment of natural history in patients treated without surgery. *Radiology* 1992;185:135.

# *Lateral Herniated Disc, Lumbar Spine*

### KEY FACTS

- Far lateral and extra foraminal disc herniations constitute 1% to 11% of all lumbar disc herniations.
- This condition implies rupture of the annulus fibrosus.
- This condition tends to occur more often among older (>50 years) male patients.
- Most far lateral herniated discs occur at the L2-3 and L3-4 levels.
- Most herniations irritate the nerve roots at the level of herniation.
- Some lateral herniated discs occasionally produce bone erosion.
- Differential diagnosis includes conjoined nerve root, perineural cysts, and neurofibroma.
- Lateral disc herniation may be a cause of the failed back syndrome.

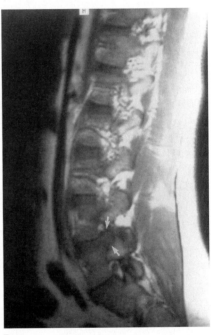

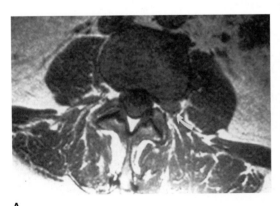

**A**                                                        **B**

**FIGURE 21-2**   (A) Axial T1-weighted MR image shows left foraminal disc herniation (*arrow*) at L3-4 level. (B) Parasagittal T1-weighted MR image of a different patient shows foraminal disc herniation (*arrows*) at L4-5. The signal intensity of the normal fat in this nerral foramen is not seen.

### Suggested Reading

Ackerman SJ, Steinberg EP, Bryan RN, BenDebba M, Long DM. Persistent low back pain patients suspected of having herniated nucleus pulposus: radiology predictors of functional outcome—implications for treatment selection. *Radiology* 1997;203:815.

# *Free Herniated Disc Fragment, Lumbar Spine*

## KEY FACTS

- A free disc fragment implies a ruptured annulus fibrosus and posterior longitudinal ligament with migration of disc fragments.
- Free disc fragments may migrate superiorly, inferiorly, or bidirectionally.
- The fragments may move into the lateral recess or posterior to the thecal sac and then become "sequestered."
- The fragments may be surrounded by granulation tissue, which enhances after administration of contrast medium, especially on magnetic resonance (MR) images.

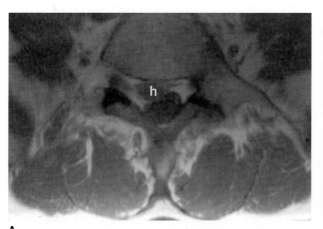

**A**

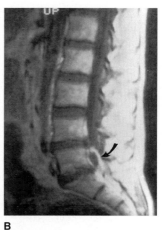

**B**

**FIGURE 21-3** **(A)** Axial postcontrast T1-weighted MR image shows free herniated disc fragment (*h*) posterior to body of L5. **(B)** Midsagittal postcontrast T1-weighted MR image of the same patient shows herniated disc (*arrow*) is not attached to any parent disc. There is peripheral disc enhancement.

### Suggested Reading
Schellinger D, Manz HJ, Vidic B, et al. Disk fragment migration. *Radiology* 1990;175:831.

# *Recurrent or Residual Herniated Disc, Lumbar Spine*

## KEY FACTS

- Recurrent or residual herniated disc is a common cause of failed back syndrome. It occurs among as many as 40% of patients after operations on the lumbar spine for disc herniation.
- This condition usually manifests itself in the immediately postoperative period.
- Caution is needed in examining patients during the initial days or weeks after the operation because the MR images may be very similar to preoperative images, and the findings do not imply failure of surgical treatment.
- MRI with contrast medium is >90% accurate in differentiating postsurgical disc herniation (does not enhance) from scar (becomes markedly enhanced). The accuracy of contrast-enhanced computed tomography (CT) is 80% or less.
- MRI should be performed immediately (<5 minutes) after administration of contrast medium. On delayed images disc herniation may become enhanced because of ingrowth of granulation tissue.

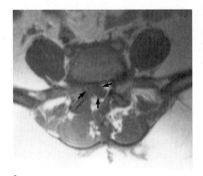 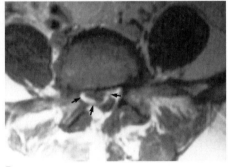

A                                  B

FIGURE 21-4    (A) Axial noncontrast T1-weighted MR image after right L5 laminotomy shows mass (*arrows*) of intermediate signal intensity. (B) Corresponding postcontrast T1-weighted image shows peripheral enhancement (*arrows*) but no enhancement in the substance of this recurrent herniated disc.

## Suggested Reading

Bundschuh CV. Imaging of the postoperative lumbosacral spine. *Neuroimaging Clin North Am* 1993;3:499.

# *Postsurgical Epidural Fibrosis, Lumbar Spine*

## KEY FACTS

- The role of epidural scarring in failed back syndrome is controversial, and the amount of scar does not correlate with clinical symptoms.

- The most important aspect of imaging is differentiating scar from recurrent or residual disc herniation (most surgeons do not perform operations for scarring).

- Less common causes of failed back syndrome include stenosis of lateral recesses, central stenosis, arachnoiditis, synovial cysts, epidural abscess, and epidural hematoma.

- Epidural fibrosis becomes enhanced after administration of contrast medium and occasionally has a mass effect.

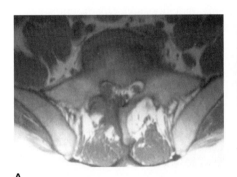 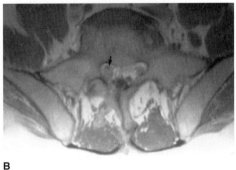

A                                    B

**FIGURE 21-5**    **(A)** Noncontrast T1-weighted MR image shows abnormal soft-tissue intensity extending from the right laminotomy into the right lateral recess. **(B)** Corresponding postcontrast T1-weighted image shows enhancement of this abnormality compatible with fibrosis. The right S1 nerve root sleeve (*arrow*) is well seen, and the distal thecal sac is retracted toward the scar.

## Suggested Reading

Dina TS, Boden SD, Davis DO. Lumbar spine after surgery of herniated disk: imaging findings in the early postoperative period. *Am J Roentgenol* 1995;164:665.

# *Isolated Enhancing Nerve Root*

### KEY FACTS

- Isolated enhancing nerve root occurs among 5% of low backs that are not treated surgically; it may be symptomatic or asymptomatic.

- This condition occurs among 21% of patients with focal lumbar disc protrusion (75% if triple-dose MR contrast medium is given).

- It may occur at multiple levels.

- This condition may imply active nerve root inflammation and breakdown of the blood-nerve barrier. Some enhancement is related to slow flow of blood through perineural venules or slow flow in the lumbar veins.

- This condition may occur after operations on the back and may be related to arachnoiditis, but 88% of cases are associated with epidural fibrosis.

- Differential diagnosis includes metastasis, Guillain-Barré syndrome, cytomegalovirus infection, lymphoma, radiation, and hypertrophic polyneuropathy (most of these result in enhancement of multiple nerve roots).

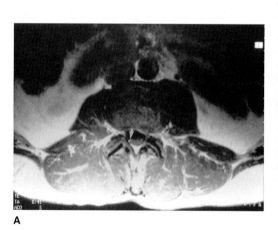
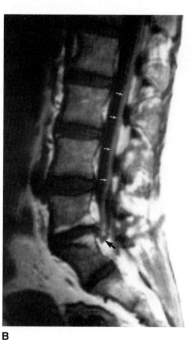

A                                         B

FIGURE 21-6    (A) Axial postcontrast T1-weighted MR image of a patient without symptoms shows enhancement (*arrow*) compatible with either a nerve root or a lumbar vein. (B) Parasagittal postcontrast T1-weighted image shows enhancement (*small arrows*) of the S1 nerve root being compressed by the herniated disc (*large arrow*).

### Suggested Reading
Itoh R, Murata K, Kamata M, Mukubou N, Morita R. Lumbosacral nerve root enhancement with disk herniation on contrast-enhanced MR. *Am J Neuroradiol* 1996;17:1619.

# *Arachnoiditis*

### KEY FACTS

- Arachnoiditis affects all three meningeal layers; therefore *arachnoiditis* is a misnomer.
- Arachnoiditis occurs among 6% to 16% of patients who have undergone spine operations but may also be seen after infections, intrathecal administration of steroids or anesthetic agents, trauma, subarachnoid hemorrhage, and myelography.
- The most common presenting symptoms are chronic pain radiating to legs, hypesthesia, paraparesis, and occasionally paraplegia.
- Different types of arachnoiditis are based on myelographic findings, as follows: (1) featureless thecal sac appearance, (2) multiple localized filling defects, nerve roots may be adherent to walls of thecal sac, and (3) soft-tissue mass filling the spinal canal (lack of enhancement at MRI suggests arachnoiditis rather than tumor).

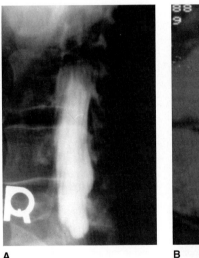

A

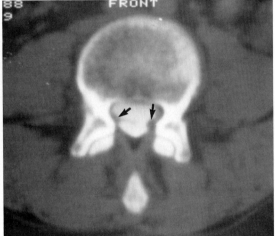

B

**FIGURE 21-7**
**(A)** Oblique view myelogram shows featureless thecal sac (nonvisualization of nerve root sleeves and distal blunting) compatible with mild arachnoiditis. **(B)** Axial postmyelographic CT scan shows empty thecal sac from adhesion of nerve roots (*arrows*) to dura. **(C)** Axial T1-weighted MR image shows marked clumping of nerve roots.

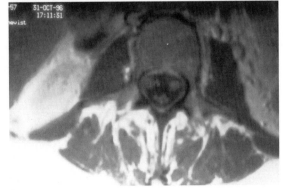

C

## Suggested Reading
Fitt GJ, Stevens JM. Postoperative arachnoiditis diagnosed by high resolution fast spin-echo MRI of the lumbar spine. *Neuroradiology* 1995;37:139.

# Synovial Cysts, Lumbar Spine

### KEY FACTS

- Synovial cyst of the lumbar spine is an uncommon entity representing protruding pouch of synovium and arising from a degenerated facet joint (may be unilateral or bilateral).
- The cyst is filled with fluid, a gelatin-like substance, blood, and/or air.
- Margins may be calcified or erode adjacent bone, and the walls occasionally become enhanced.
- Most cysts occur at the L3-5 levels (75% at L4).
- The cysts generally present with radiculopathy.
- Differential diagnosis is ganglion cysts.
- On T2-weighted MR images, the adjacent facet joint may show increased signal intensity in the intraarticular space because of effusion caused by degenerative changes.

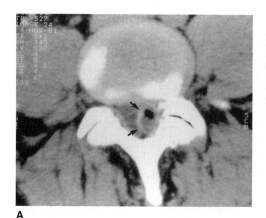 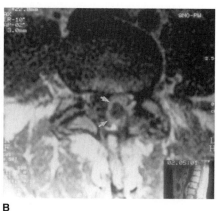

A                B

**FIGURE 21-8**    **(A)** Axial CT scan shows mass (*arrows*) adjacent to left L4-5 facet joint. There is gas in this cyst and in the adjacent facet joint. **(B)** Axial postcontrast T1-weighted MR image of a different patient shows left-sided synovial cyst at L4-5 with peripheral enhancement (*arrows*).

## Suggested Reading

Gorey MT, Hayman RA, Black KS, et al. Lumbar synovial cysts eroding bone. *Am J Neuro-radiol* 1993;13:161.

# *Spondylolysis and Spondylolisthesis, Lumbar Spine*

## KEY FACTS

*   *Spondylolysis* is a cleft (with fibrous union) of one or both pars interarticularis of a vertebra; the most common levels are L5 and L4. Most clefts are bilateral. They may be congenital or posttraumatic in nature, are found in 1% to 5% of population, and are better seen on oblique plain radiographs, axial CT scans, and far lateral sagittal MR images.

*   *Spondylolisthesis* refers to displacement (posterior or anterior) of a vertebra with respect to adjacent ones. It may be caused by ligamentous laxity associated with degenerative changes or by spondylolysis (especially among young persons) or be a sequela of trauma; L4 through S1 are the most common levels. On midsagittal MR images the anteroposterior diameter of the spinal canal is widened in spondylolisthesis caused by spondylolysis but not in cases caused by degenerative facet disease.

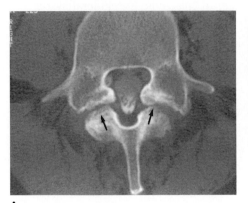 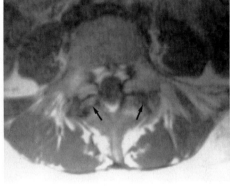

**A**  **B**

**FIGURE 21-9**  (A) Axial postmyelographic CT scan shows bilateral pars interarticularis defects (*arrows*). The diameter of the thecal sac is elongated in its antero-posterior dimension. (B) Corresponding axial T1-weighted MR image of the same patient shows the defects (*arrows*).

## Suggested Reading

Ulmer JL, Elster AD, Mathews VP, King JC. Distinction between degenerative and isthmic spondylolisthesis on sagittal MR images: importance of increased anteroposterior diameter of the spinal canal (wide canal sign). *Am J Roentgenol* 1994;163:411.

# *Herniated Disc, Cervical Spine*

## KEY FACTS

- Herniation of a disc in the cervical spine may be symptomatic or asymptomatic. Most occur during the fourth or fifth decades of life. There is no history of trauma in most instances, but herniation may be caused by trauma.
- At MRI degenerative changes in the cervical spine are present in 25% of the population younger than 40 years and in 60% of population older than 60 years.
- Most frequently involved levels are C5-6 (30%) and C6-7 (60%).
- MRI with surface coil is as sensitive as postmyelographic CT for detection of cervical herniated discs.
- Axial MR images have to be T2-weighted to depict white cerebrospinal fluid (CSF) and provide contrast with adjacent bone (addition of magnetization transfer increases conspicuity of disc herniations); T1-weighted imaging may be performed after administration of gadolinium (contrast is then produced by means of enhancing the epidural plexus against black bone and CSF).

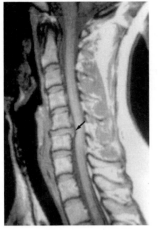

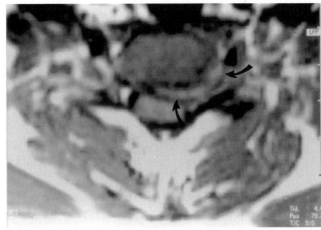

A                              B

**FIGURE 21-10**
**(A)** Midsagittal T1-weighted MR image shows herniated disc (*arrow*) at C5-6 producing compression of the spinal cord. **(B)** Axial T1-weighted MR image of a different patient shows herniated disc (*arrows*) compressing the spinal cord and extending into the left neural foramen. **(C)** Axial gradient echo (T2*)–weighted image shows disc herniation (*arrow*) in left C5-6 neural foramen.

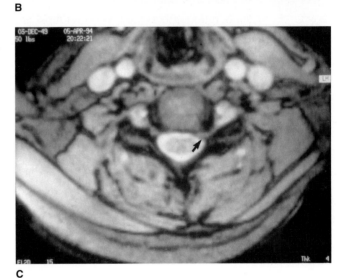

C

## Suggested Reading

Finelli DA, Hurst GC, Karaman BA, Simon JE, Duerk JL, Bellon EM. Use of magnetization transfer for improved contrast on gradient-echo MR images of the cervical spine. *Radiology* 1994;193:165.

# *Ossified Posterior Longitudinal Ligament*

### KEY FACTS

- Ossification of the posterior longitudinal ligament is most common in Japan, where it affects 2% to 4% of the population, generally persons between 60 and 70 years of age.
- This condition represents heterotopic bone formation caused by repeated mechanical stress.
- The condition is associated with diffuse idiopathic skeletal hyperostosis (DISH).
- Ossification can be continuous or segmental and may produce spinal cord compression (in general, cervical spinal canal stenosis occurs with an anteroposterior diameter <12 mm).
- The condition affects the C4-6 level most commonly.

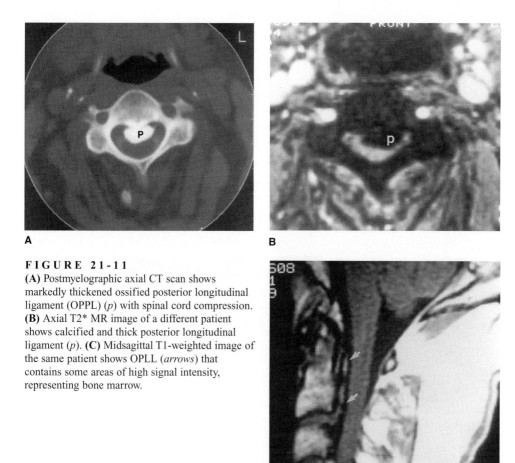

**A**

**B**

**C**

**FIGURE 21-11**
**(A)** Postmyelographic axial CT scan shows markedly thickened ossified posterior longitudinal ligament (OPPL) (*p*) with spinal cord compression. **(B)** Axial T2* MR image of a different patient shows calcified and thick posterior longitudinal ligament (*p*). **(C)** Midsagittal T1-weighted image of the same patient shows OPLL (*arrows*) that contains some areas of high signal intensity, representing bone marrow.

## Suggested Reading
Otake S, Marsuo M, Nishizawa S, et al. Ossification of the posterior longitudinal ligament: MR evaluation. *Am J Neuroradiol* 1992;13:1059.

# *Thoracic Disc Herniation*

### KEY FACTS

- Thoracic disc herniation is less common than disc herniation in the cervical and lumbar regions; most occur in the middle to lower thoracic regions.

- Small herniations are asymptomatic; large ones result in myelopathy (correct clinical diagnosis is made for less than 50% of patients).

- Most lesions are of low signal intensity with both T1- and T2-weighted sequences.

- On CT scans, many thoracic herniations show an area of bone sclerosis in the adjacent vertebral end plates (nuclear tail or trail).

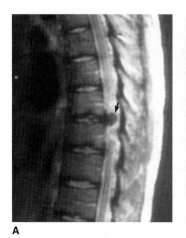

**A**

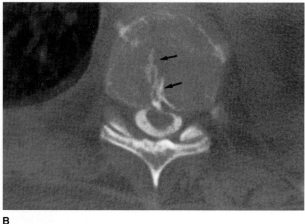

**B**

FIGURE 21-12    **(A)** Midsagittal T2-weighted MR image shows hypointense herniated disc (*arrow*) in midthoracic region resulting in considerable compression of the spinal cord. **(B)** Axial CT scan (after myelography) of a patient with a small thoracic disc herniation shows nuclear trail (*arrows*).

### Suggested Reading

Awwad EE, Martin DS, Smith KR. The nuclear trial sign in thoracic herniated disks. *Am J Neuroradiol* 1992;13:137.

# 22 Tumors and Tumor-Like Conditions

## *Vertebral Body Metastases*

### KEY FACTS

- Vertebral metastases occur in 5% to 10% of all patients with cancer, especially those with primary tumors of the breast, prostate, uterus, lung, or myeloma or lymphoma.
- Most metastases have a combined osseous-epidural-intradural location.
- Most metastases occur in the thoracic spine.
- Metastases are multiple among 90% of patients.
- The most common symptoms of metastases include pain, weakness, autonomic dysfunction, and sensory loss.
- Most vertebral body metastases may be screened with noncontrast sagittal T1-weighted magnetic resonance (MR) images. Evaluation of epidural-intradural extension requires administration of contrast medium. After administration of contrast medium, most vertebral metastases become isointense to normal marrow and difficult to visualize (fat suppression may be needed in this situation).
- Diffusion-weighted MR imaging may be helpful in differentiating pathologic vertebral compression fractures from osteoporotic ones. Pathologic compression fractures are hyperintense.

*(continued)*

## *Vertebral Body Metastases* (Continued)

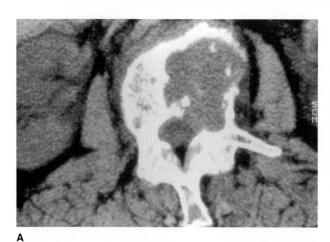

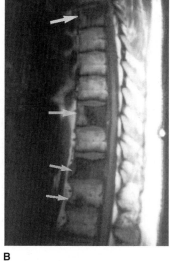

A

B

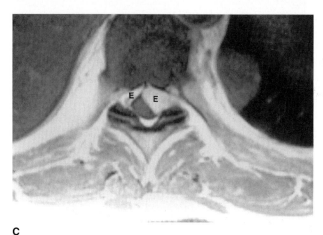

C

**FIGURE 22-1**
(A) Axial CT scan shows lytic lesion affecting a lumbar vertebral body and left pedicle. Primary tumor was renal cell adenocarcinoma. (B) Noncontrast midsagittal T1-weighted MR image shows zones of low signal intensity (*arrows*) in multiple vertebrae. These metastases were from breast carcinoma. (C) Postcontrast axial T1-weighted MR image (different patient) shows metastasis in the ventral epidural space (*E*). The abnormality has a "curtain" appearance because it drapes over the midline fibrous septum.

### Suggested Reading

Baur A, Stäbler A, Brüning R, et al. Diffusion-weighted MR imaging of bone marrow: differentiation of benign versus pathologic compression fractures. *Radiology* 1998;207:349.

# Sequelae of Irradiation

## KEY FACTS

- After irradiation, T1-weighted MR images show high signal intensity (fatty replacement of bone marrow) in vertebral bodies corresponding to port.

- Radiation myelitis occurs among 2% to 3% of patients generally 12 to 24 months after treatment. It is probably related to vasculitis. It is manifested by increased T2 signal intensity, increased thickness of the spinal cord, and absence of contrast enhancement.

- Radiation also may induce a neuritis.

- There is an increased risk (very small) for development of secondary sarcomas.

- If radiation treatment is given before an operation, there is 36% risk for postoperative infection.

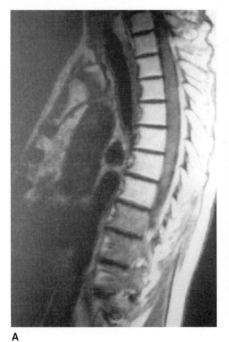 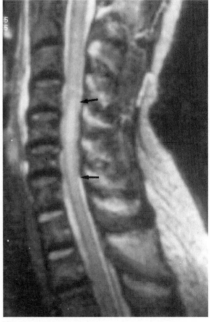

A          B

**FIGURE 22-2**     **(A)** Midsagittal noncontrast T1-weighted MR image shows increased signal intensity in the marrow of the mid-to-upper thoracic vertebral bodies corresponding to radiation port. **(B)** T2-weighted image of a different patient after radiation treatment for laryngeal cancer shows increased signal intensity (*arrows*) from C4 to C7 that suggests radiation myelitis.

## Suggested Reading

Valk PE, Dillon WP. Radiation Injury to the Brain. *Am J Neuroradiol* 1991;12:45.

# *Spinal Cord and Leptomeningeal Metastases*

KEY FACTS

- Spinal cord and leptomeningeal metastases occur among less than 1% of patients with cancer, especially those with primary tumors of the lung (>50%) and breast or those with lymphoma, melanoma, colorectal carcinoma, head and neck carcinoma, or leukemia.

- The thoracic spinal cord is most commonly involved.

- Although secondary to hematogenous dissemination, spinal cord metastases from primary central nervous system (CNS) tumors (mainly medulloblastoma) spread along cerebrospinal fluid (CSF) pathways.

- Metastasis may involve the leptomeninges, but concomitant bone disease is uncommon.

- Tumors outside the CNS that may produce CSF spread include breast carcinoma, lung carcinoma, melanoma, gastrointestinal tract carcinoma, and lymphoma, but metastasis also occurs among as many as 50% of patients with lymphoblastic or myelogenous leukemia.

- Tumors of the CNS that most commonly spread through the CSF include medulloblastoma, ependymoma, and glioma.

- Faint enhancement along the ventral surface of the conus medullaris may be normal vascular enhancement and should not be confused with metastases; enhancement also may occur 4 to 6 weeks after operations on the spine or posterior fossa.

- The most common sites of leptomeningeal metastases in the spine are lumbar, thoracic, and cervical regions.

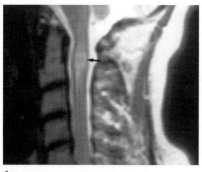
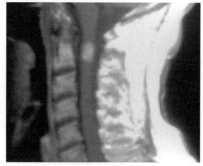

**A**                                    **B**

**FIGURE 22-3**
**(A)** Midsagittal T2-weighted MR image of a patient with primary breast cancer shows bright lesion (*arrow*) at the C2 level. **(B)** Corresponding postcontrast T1-weighted image shows enhancement of intramedullary metastasis. **(C)** Postcontrast midsagittal T1-weighted MR image of a different patient shows intramedullary and pial metastases in the conus medullaris (*open arrows*) and in one lumbar nerve root (*solid arrow*).

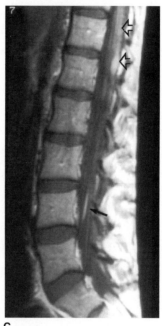

**C**

## Suggested Reading

Post Donovan MJ, Quencer RM, Green BA, et al. Intramedullary spinal cord metastases, mainly of nonneurogenic origin. *Am J Neuroradiol* 1987;8:339.

# Spinal Cord Astrocytoma

## KEY FACTS

- More than 75% of instances of spinal cord astrocytoma (among both children and adults) have low-grade histologic features. This tumor occurs more often among men.
- This is the second most common primary spinal cord tumor after ependymoma.
- Most spinal cord astrocytomas involve the cervicothoracic region.
- Most are discovered during the third and fourth decades of life.
- Early symptoms are nonspecific or nonlocalizing and include pain and scoliosis.
- The tumor is slow growing and causes bone changes in 50% of instances.
- Associated cysts are common (40%), and holocord involvement is not rare.
- Almost all spinal cord astrocytomas become enhanced on postcontrast MR images.

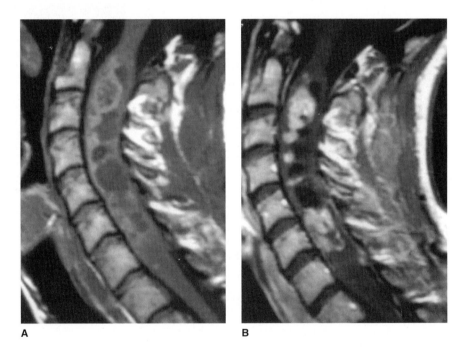

A                                                 B

**FIGURE 22-4**   **(A)** Noncontrast midsagittal T1-weighted MR image shows a nonhomogeneous astrocytoma involving the spinal cord from C2 to T1. **(B)** Corresponding postcontrast T2-weighted image shows enhancement of several tumor nodules. (Courtesy M. Smith, M.D., Nashville, TN)

## Suggested Reading

Nemoto Y, Inoue Y, Tashiro T, et al. Intramedullary spinal cord tumors: significance of associated hemorrhage at MR imaging. *Radiology* 1992;182:793.

# Spinal Cord Ependymoma

KEY FACTS

- Spinal cord ependymoma is the most common (65%) primary tumor of the spinal cord.
- It occurs predominantly in the lower spinal cord, conus medullaris, and filum terminale (at this location it is typically of the myxopapillary subtype, and the differential diagnosis includes astrocytoma and paraganglioma).
- The tumor is found during the fifth and sixth decades of life with a slight female predominance.
- The tumor typically presents with only back pain, but occasionally patients have leg weakness and sphincter dysfunction.
- Spinal cord ependymoma is associated with neurofibromatosis type 2; all tumors are slow growing and may produce bone scalloping; widening of the spinal canal occurs in 30% of instances.
- About 64% of patients have evidence of prior hemorrhage on MR images. Images show well-defined margins (although occasionally they invade the conus medullaris), and all become enhanced after administration of MR contrast medium.
- Intratumoral cysts are more common than with astrocytoma.

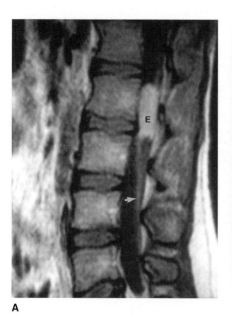 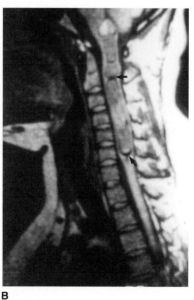

A        B

FIGURE 22-5    **(A)** Postcontrast midsagittal T1-weighted MR image shows a myxopapillary ependymoma (*E*) in the filum terminale. The distal filum terminale (*arrow*) became enhanced and was found at operation to be infiltrated by tumor. **(B)** Precontrast midsagittal T1-weighted MR image of a different patient shows ependymoma of the cervicomedullary region. The tumor contains several hypointense areas (*arrows*) suggesting old blood products.

## Suggested Reading

Kahan H, Sklar EM, Post MJD, Bruce JH. MR characteristics of histopathologic subtypes of spinal ependymomas. *Am J Neuroradiol* 1996;17:143.

# *Spinal Schwannoma and Meningioma*

KEY FACTS

- Schwannoma neurofibroma are the most common spinal tumors; meningioma is second (25%).
- Both are most likely histologically benign and are found among middle-aged (40 to 60 years) women.
- Most nerve sheath tumors are found in the cervical region; meningiomas occur in the thoracic (80%), cervical (15%), and lumbar (5%) regions.
- Most nerve sheath tumors are both extradural and intradural (dumbbell shaped), whereas most meningiomas are entirely intradural and lateral to the spinal cord.
- At computed tomography (CT), 10% of meningiomas show calcifications. Nerve sheath tumors may show a target appearance after administration of contrast medium and are occasionally cystic or hemorrhagic.
- Spinal neurofibromas are more common among patients with neurofibromatosis type 1; schwannomas occur in neurofibromatosis type 2 and among patients without this disease.
- Malignant degeneration of neurofibroma occurs among 4% to 11% of patients with neurofibromatosis type 1; malignant degeneration of schwannomas is extremely rare.

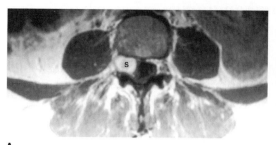

A

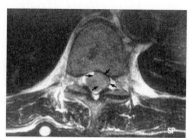

B

## FIGURE 22-6

**(A)** Axial postcontrast T1-weighted MR image shows enhancing right-sided lumbar schwannoma (*S*) expanding the neural foramen. **(B)** Axial postcontrast T1-weighted MR image of a different patient shows extramedullary thoracic meningioma (*arrows*). **(C)** Midsagittal postcontrast T1-weighted MR image of a different patient shows intraspinal thoracic meningioma (*arrow*). Note incidental old compression fracture in midthoracic region.

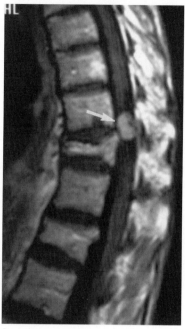

C

## Suggested Reading

Matsumoto S, Hasu K, Uchino A, et al. MR of intradural-extramedullary spinal neurinomas and meningiomas. *Clin Imaging* 1993;17:46.

# *Vertebral Body Hemangioma*

KEY FACTS

- Vertebral body hemangioma occurs among 11% of the population. Most are solitary (70%), although about 30% are multiple. The most common locations include the thoracic and lumbar spine. This lesion is more common among women.

- Most vertebral body hemangiomas never produce symptoms, but occasionally they may lead to spinal cord compression.

- Most show high signal intensity on T1-weighted MR images and may continue to have slightly high signal intensity on T2-weighted images (remember that focal fatty deposits also are bright on fast spin echo T2-weighted MR images).

- Occasional aggressive hemangiomas show lower signal intensity on both T1- (less fat) and T2-weighted MR images and may be indistinguishable from metastases.

- On CT scans and plain films, thick bone trabeculae (corduroy pattern) are typical.

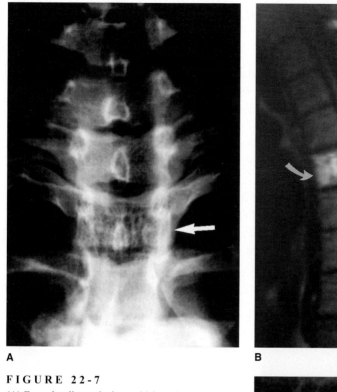

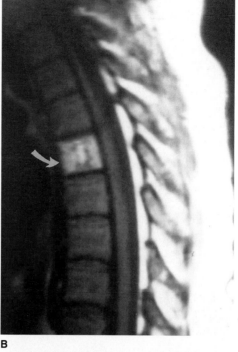

## FIGURE 22-7

(A) Frontal radiograph shows thickened secondary trabeculae caused by hemangioma in the vertebral body of T1 (*arrow*). (B) Noncontrast midsagittal T1-weighted MR image of a different patient shows bright signal intensity from a hemangioma (*arrow*) involving a midthoracic vertebral body. (C) Axial noncontrast T2-weighted image of the same patient shows bright hemangioma with focal areas of hypointensity caused by thick trabeculae or blood vessels.

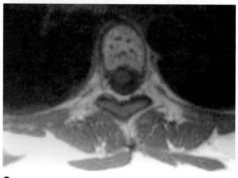

## Suggested Reading

Laredo JD, Assouline E, Gelbert F, et al. Vertebral hemangiomas: fat content as a sign of aggressiveness. *Radiology* 1990;177:467.

# Aneurysmal Bone Cyst

### KEY FACTS

- Aneurysmal bone cysts (ABCs) constitute less than 2% of primary bone tumors of the spine and are histologically benign but locally aggressive.
- About 20% of all ABCs occur in the spine, and the neural arch is more commonly (60%) involved than the vertebral bodies (40%).
- It is believed that many ABCs arise from other underlying lesions such as chondroblastoma, giant cell tumor, osteoblastoma, and fibroosseous lesions.
- ABCs generally are discovered in adolescents and present with pain, paraplegia, mass, and radicular symptoms.
- ABCs are expansile masses with a thin rim of bone and on MR images and CT scans have a complex appearance as the result of repeated intratumoral hemorrhaging.

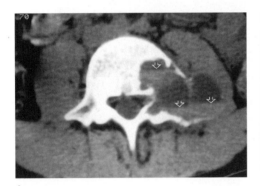 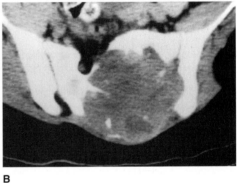

A                                                          B

FIGURE 22-8    (A) Axial CT scan shows aneurysmal bone cyst involving L4. Note expansion of bone, extension into the left psoas muscle, and blood levels (*arrows*). (B) Axial CT scan of a different patient shows solid aneurysmal bone cyst involving the sacrum.

### Suggested Reading

Munk PL, Helms CA, Holt RG, et al. MR imaging of aneurysmal bone cysts. *Am J Roentgenol* 1989;153:99.

# Giant Cell Tumor

KEY FACTS

- Giant cell tumor constitutes 4% to 5% of all primary bone tumors, and only 7% are found in the spine.
- The most common locations in the spine are the sacrum and the thoracic, cervical, and lumbar regions.
- Malignant degeneration occurs among 5% to 10% of these tumors.
- The tumor tends to involve the vertebral body (with superimposed fracture the tumor may produce compression of the spinal cord) and contains blood.
- Recurrences after surgical treatment occur among 40% to 60% of patients.

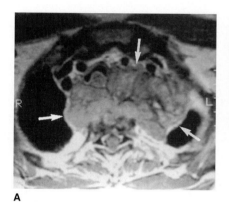 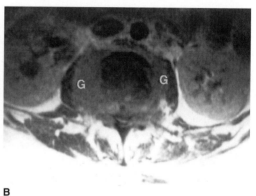

A                                           B

**FIGURE 22-9**      **(A)** Axial postcontrast T1-weighted MR image shows large and enhancing giant cell tumor (GCT, *arrows*) arising from an upper thoracic vertebral body. There is anterior displacement of the mediastinal structures. **(B)** Noncontrast axial CT scan of a different patient shows large soft-tissue mass (*G*) at L2 level extending into the spinal canal and compressing the thecal sac. At biopsy, this was found to be a GCT.

## Suggested Reading

Meyers SP, Yaw K, Devaney K. Giant cell tumor of the thoracic spine: MR appearance. *Am J Neuroradiol* 1994;15:962.

# Osteoid Osteoma

### KEY FACTS

- Osteoid osteoma constitutes 10% of all primary bone tumors, and 10% of them are found in the spine.

- Most are found among boys 6 to 17 years of age.

- The most common locations are the lumbar (60%), cervical (27%), thoracic (12%), and sacral (1%) regions.

- Most arise in the pedicles, laminae, facet joints, and spinous processes.

- Most result in pain (worse at night), radiculopathy, gait abnormalities, scoliosis, and muscle atrophy.

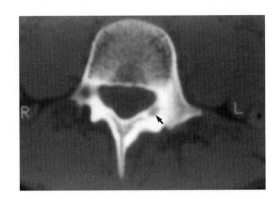

**FIGURE 22-10**

Axial CT scan shows a thick and sclerotic left lamina and pedicle of L3. Note central lucent nidus (*arrow*).

## Suggested Reading

Assoun J, Richardi G, Railhac JJ, et al. Osteoid osteoma: MR imaging versus CT. *Radiology* 1994;191:217.

# Eosinophilic Granuloma

**KEY FACTS**

- Eosinophilic granuloma is the localized and most common (70%) form of histiocytosis of Langerhans (histiocytosis X).
- Common sites of involvement are the skull, mandible, spine, ribs, femur, and humerus.
- In the spine this tumor predominantly affects the vertebral body, and mechanical stress results in a vertebra plana. The discs are preserved, and very little soft-tissue mass is associated with this tumor.

*(continued)*

# *Eosinophilic Granuloma (Continued)*

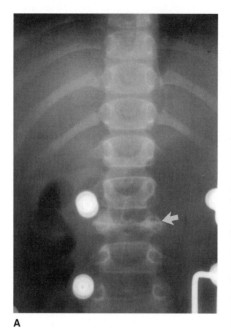

**A**

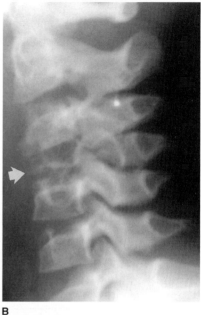

**B**

**FIGURE 22-11**

(A) Frontal radiograph shows L3 vertebra plana (*arrow*). (B) Lateral radiograph shows C4 vertebra plana (*arrow*). (C) Midsagittal T2-weighted MR image of a different patient shows nearly complete collapse of an upper thoracic vertebral body (*arrow*). No soft-tissue mass is associated with the lesion.

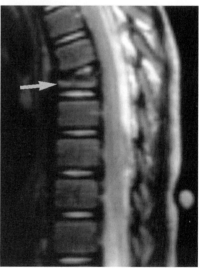

**C**

## Suggested Reading

De Schepper AM, Ramon F, Van Marck E. MR imaging of eosinophilic granuloma: report of 11 cases. *Skeletal Radiol* 1993;22:163.

# *Chordoma*

### KEY FACTS

- Chordomas arise from notochordal remnants at the sacrum (50%) (most common primary sacral tumor), clivus (35%), and cervical and thoracic regions (15%).

- They are locally aggressive; metastases occur among 10% to 40% of patients.

- Chordoma generally occurs among men between the fifth and seventh decades of life, although vertebral body chordomas occur earlier in life.

- The tumor is usually a lytic and destructive lesion that presents with pain, rectal dysfunction, mass, and urinary incontinence.

- CT shows that 30% to 70% of these tumors contain calcifications.

- Most chordomas are of relatively low signal intensity on T2-weighted MR images, but the chondroid type may show relatively high signal intensity on T2-weighted MR images.

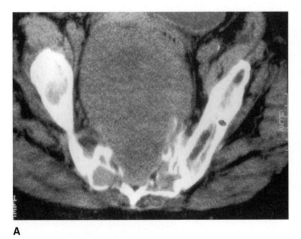

**A**

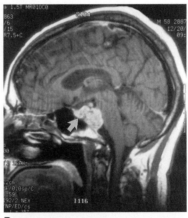

**B**

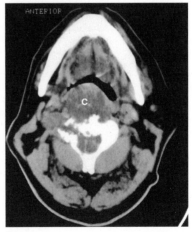

**C**

**FIGURE 22-12**

**(A)** Axial CT scan shows large soft-tissue mass arising from and destroying the sacrum. **(B)** Midsagittal postcontrast T1-weighted MR image of a different patient shows clival chondroid chordoma (*arrow*). Unlike this tumor, most chordomas in this region destroy the clivus. **(C)** Axial CT scan of a different patient shows a chordoma (*c*) arising from and destroying C2.

## Suggested Reading
Weber AL, Liebsch NJ, Sanchez R, Sweriduc ST. Chordomas of the skull base: radiologic and clinical evaluation. *Neuroimaging Clin North Am* 1994;4:515.

# Paget's Disease

### KEY FACTS

- Paget's disease affects 3% of population older than 40 years.
- The disease may have a solitary location or involve multiple bones.
- Multiple sites include mainly the spine (75%), skull (65%), and pelvis (40%).
- The most common symptoms include pain, motor weakness, incontinence, and cord compression (from superimposed fractures).
- In the initial *osteolytic phase,* MR images show fibrous conversion of marrow, which contains multiple enlarged vessels; these changes disappear in the *mixed phase,* and finally, in the *osteosclerotic phase,* the bone marrow returns to normal, and bone cortices are thickened.
- New onset of pain in a bone involved in Paget's disease should raise the possibility of sarcomatous degeneration.

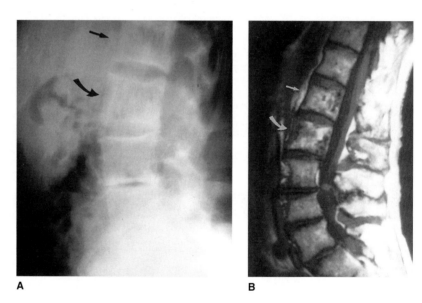

A                                                    B

**FIGURE  22-13**    **(A)** Lateral radiograph shows Paget's disease involving L3 (*curved arrow*) and L2 (*straight arrow*). **(B)** Midsagittal T1-weighted MR image of the same patient shows mottled signal intensity in L3 (*curved arrow*) and L2 (*straight arrow*). The affected vertebrae appear slightly enlarged.

### Suggested Reading
Roberts MC, Kressel HY, Fallon MD, et al. Paget disease: MR imaging findings. *Radiology* 1989;173:341.

# *Spinal Cord Cyst*

**KEY FACTS**

- *Hydromyelia* is dilatation of the central canal, and *syringomyelia* is a spinal cord cavity separate from the central canal; it is not clinically important to differentiate between the two types of cyst.

- Most cysts are congenital (associated with the Chiari I and II malformations), posttraumatic, or secondary to tumors.

- They occur at any location, but congenital cysts tend to be more common in the cervical and upper thoracic regions.

- They may occur above or below the level of prior trauma.

- The most common symptoms include pain and temperature alterations, weakness followed by atrophy, motor disturbances, spastic paraparesis, and neurotrophic joints (especially the shoulder and elbow).

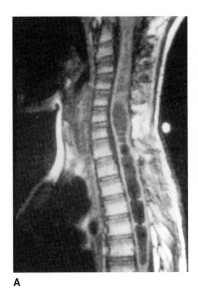 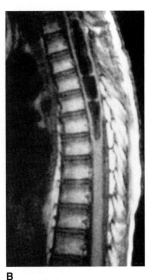

A                                    B

**FIGURE 22-14**    **(A)** Midsagittal noncontrast T1-weighted MR image shows multiseptated spinal cord cyst involving the cervicothoracic region. **(B)** Midsagittal noncontrast T1-weighted MR image of the same patient shows the lower extent of the spinal cord cyst.

## Suggested Reading

Kochan PJ, Quencer RM. Imaging of cystic and cavitary lesions of the spinal cord and canal. *Radiol Clin North Am* 1991;29:867.

# Perineural (Tarlov) Cyst

## KEY FACTS

- Perineural cysts arise at the junction of the posterior nerve roots and nerve ganglia between the endoneurium and perineurium.
- They are most common in the sacrum (S2 and S3) but may be found at any level in the spine.
- The cysts may be solitary or multiple.
- They may communicate freely with the subarachnoid space (and therefore opacify immediately during myelography), have partial communication (therefore fill slowly after myelography), or be noncommunicating and expand owing to a ball-valve mechanism that traps CSF.
- If expansile, perineural cysts may produce pain as nerve roots traveling along the margins of the cyst become compressed.
- Differential diagnosis includes epidermoid, intrasacral meningocele, and dural ectasia secondary to neurofibromatosis type 1 or collagen disorders, such as Marfan's syndrome.

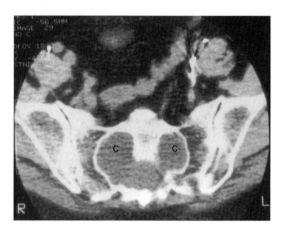

**FIGURE 22-15**
Axial CT scan shows expansion of expansile nerve root sleeve cysts (*C*) in the sacrum.

## Suggested Reading

Paulsen RD, Call GA, Murtagh FR. Prevalence and percutaneous drainage of cysts of the sacral nerve root sheath (Tarlov cysts). *Am J Neuroradiol* 1994;15:293.

# *Epidural Lipomatosis*

### KEY FACTS

- Epidural lipomatosis represents hypertrophy of normal and nonencapsulated epidural fat as the result of large body habitus, exogenous steroid administration, or Cushing's disease.
- The most common locations are the thoracic (posterior) and lumbar spine (concentric).
- The lesions may cause chronic nonspecific back pain or even myelopathy.
- Differential diagnosis includes epidural hematoma (which has an acute onset of symptoms) and epidural angiolipoma.

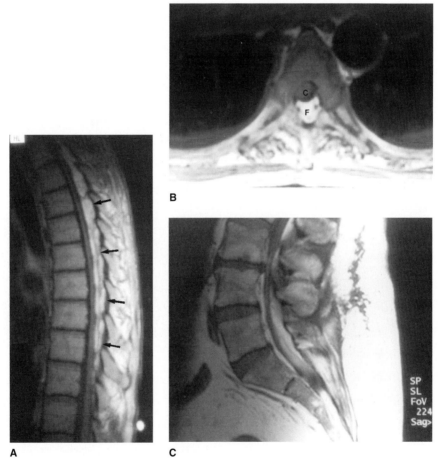

### FIGURE 22-16

**(A)** Midsagittal T1-weighted MR image shows large amount of fat (*arrows*) in the posterior thoracic epidural space. The spinal cord is diffusely thin. **(B)** Axial T1-weighted MR image of the same patient shows posterior epidural fat (*F*) displacing the spinal cord (*C*) anteriorly. **(C)** Midsagittal T1-weighted MR image of a different patient shows epidural lipomatosis in the lumbosacral region.

### Suggested Reading

Hierholzer J, Beendorf G, Lehman T, et al. Epidural lipomatosis: case report and literature review. *Neuroradiology* 1996;38:343.

# 23    Vascular Disorders

## *Spinal Cord Cavernous Angioma*

### KEY FACTS

- At histologic examination spinal cord cavernous angioma is found to be composed of dilated vascular sinusoids devoid of smooth muscle and elastic fibers. There are no normal intervening neural tissues, and abundant hemosiderin is present.
- Cavernous angiomas constitute 5% to 10% of spinal vascular malformations.
- If strictly intramedullary, angioma is usually solitary.
- Common clinical symptoms include progressive paraparesis, sensory alterations, pain, and occasionally subarachnoid hemorrhage or hematomyelia.

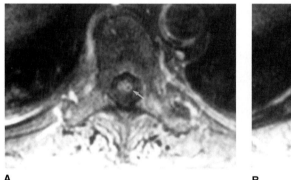
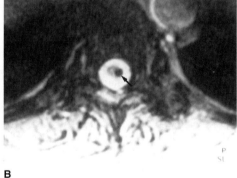

A                                    B

**FIGURE 23-1**    **(A)** Axial postcontrast T1-weighted MR image shows small and mildly enhancing lesion (*arrow*) in the left lateral aspect of the lower thoracic spinal cord. **(B)** Axial T2-weighted image shows blooming of this presumed cavernous angioma because of the presence of hemosiderin.

### Suggested Reading

Friedman DP, Flanders AE, Tartaglino LM. Vascular neoplasms and malformations, ischemia, and hemorrhage affecting the spinal cord: MR imaging findings. *Am J Roentgenol* 1994; 162:685.

# *Spinal Cord Vascular Malformations*

## KEY FACTS

- *Type 1:* a dural fistula with one single feeding artery arising from the intercostal or lumbar arteries and draining into an enlarged vein located on the dorsal surface of spinal cord; it is generally found among men 40 to 60 years of age who may have a history of spinal trauma.

- *Type 2:* a small mass-like vascular nidus (glomus) supplied by multiple feeders from anterior or posterior spinal arteries or both and draining into enlarged veins.

- *Type 3:* a large mass-like vascular nidus with extramedullary extension supplied by a myriad of arterial feeders (juvenile type).

- *Type 4:* a large malformation involving the spinal cord and adjacent vertebrae and soft tissues (metameric type).

- The most common locations are the cervical spine (type 2) and lower thoracic and upper lumbar spine (type 1); most type 2 malformations occur among middle-aged men.

- The most common symptoms include paresis, sensory alterations, autonomic dysfunction, and impotence.

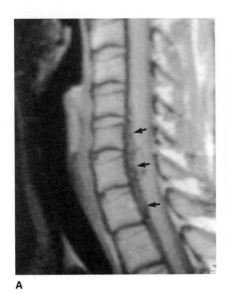 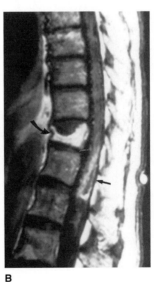

A                                      B

**FIGURE 23-2**   **(A)** Midsagittal proton-density MR image shows a myriad of flow void defects (*arrows*) in the anterior subarachnoid space and spinal cord in the midcervical region. This patient had a type 3 malformation. **(B)** Postcontrast T1-weighted MR image of a patient with a dural fistula shows enhancement (*straight arrow*) of the conus medullaris, multiple large vessels on the surface of the spinal cord, and a prior compression and enhancing fracture of a lower thoracic vertebral body (*curved arrow*).

## Suggested Reading

Hasuo K, Mizushima A, Mihara F, et al. Contrast-enhanced MRI in spinal arteriovenous malformations and fistulae before and after embolization therapy. *Neuroradiology* 1996;38:609.

# Spinal Cord Infarction

### KEY FACTS

- The most common causes of arterial spinal cord infarction include atherosclerosis, hypertension, diabetes, thoracoabdominal aortic aneurysms, sickle cell anemia, spinal trauma, caisson disease, and arteritis.
- Arterial infarction has an acute onset.
- The most common causes of venous infarction include dural arteriovenous fistula, hypercoagulable states, and fibrocartilaginous emboli.
- Venous infarction has an insidious onset and should be differentiated from subacute necrotizing myelopathy.

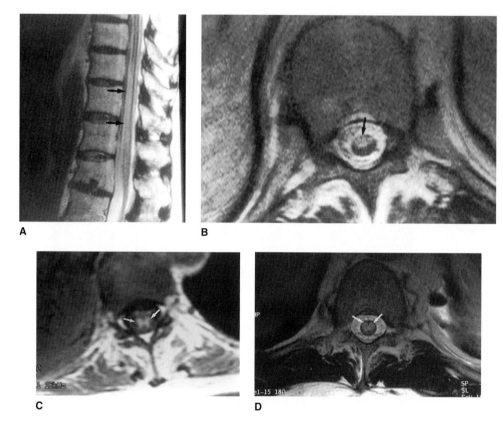

A   B

C   D

**FIGURE 23-3**   **(A)** Midsagittal T2-weighted MR image shows increased signal intensity (*arrows*) in the ventral aspect of the distal spinal cord. **(B)** Axial T2-weighted MR image of the same patient shows hyperintensity (*arrow*) in the anterior two thirds of the spinal cord. **(C)** Postcontrast axial T1-weighted MR image of a different patient shows enhancement of the gray matter in the distal spinal cord (*arrows*). **(D)** T2-weighted MR image of a different patient shows swollen and hyperintense anterior columns of gray matter (*arrows*, owl eye sign).

### Suggested Reading

Mawad ME, Rivera V, Crawford S, et al. Spinal cord ischemia after resection of thoracoabdominal aortic aneurysm: MR findings in 24 patients. *Am J Neuroradiol* 1990;11:987.

# Spinal Epidural and Subdural Hematoma

## KEY FACTS

- Spinal epidural hematoma is more common than subdural hematoma.
- Predisposing factors are coagulopathy, trauma, prior spinal puncture, spinal vascular malformations, hypertension, pregnancy, infection, advanced age, operation on the spine, forceful sneezing, and lupus erythematosus (but nearly 50% of hematomas are spontaneous).
- The most common locations are the thoracic, lumbar, and cervical regions.
- Most hematomas occur among men 40 to 60 years of age.
- Most result in symptoms caused by compression of the spinal cord.

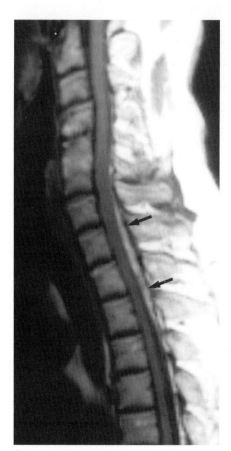

**A**

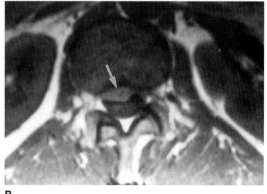

**B**

**FIGURE 23-4**  **(A)** Midsagittal noncontrast T1-weighted MR image shows epidural hematoma (*arrows*) in the posterior cervicothoracic region. **(B)** Axial T1-weighted MR image of a different patient shows biconvex epidural hematoma (*arrow*) in the ventral lumbar region. *(continued)*

# *Spinal Epidural and Subdural Hematoma*
## *(Continued)*

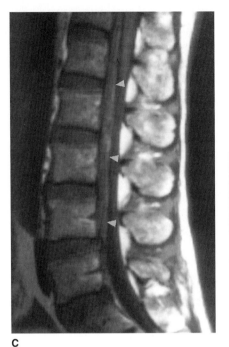

C

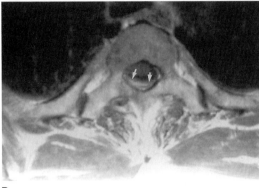

D

**FIGURE 23-4**
**CONTINUED**

**(C)** Midsagittal T1-weighted MR image of the same patient as in **B** shows complete extension of the hematoma (*arrowheads*) in the ventral epidural space. **(D)** Axial T1-weighted MR image of a different patient shows crescent-shaped dorsal thoracic subdural hematoma (*arrows*).

## Suggested Reading

Post MJD, Becerra JL, Madsen PW, et al. Acute spinal subdural hematoma: MR and CT findings with pathologic correlates. *Am J Neuroradiol* 1995;15:1895.

# 24 Inflammation and Infection

## *Ankylosing Spondylitis*

KEY FACTS

- Ankylosing spondylitis occurs among young men and is associated with histocompatibility antigen B27.
- This condition occurs among 1.4% of population.
- Sacroilitis often is the first manifestation, followed by ankylosis of the lumbar and thoracic spine, atlantoaxial subluxation, fractures, and spontaneous epidural hematoma.
- Cauda equina syndrome may occur.
- Destruction of a disc space with no underlying infection occurs among 3% to 28% of patients.
- Adherent arachnoiditis may cause bone erosion.

*(continued)*

## *Ankylosing Spondylitis (Continued)*

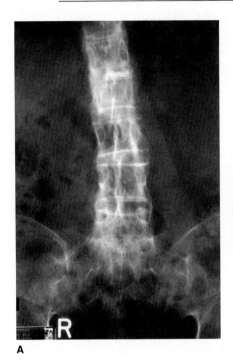

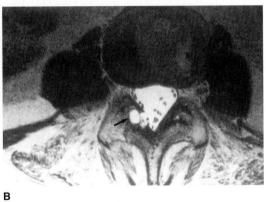

A                                B

**FIGURE 24-1**    (A) Frontal radiograph shows osteopenia, squaring of the vertebrae, and thin, bridging syndesmophytes. **(B)** Axial T2-weighted MR image of a different patient shows erosive diverticula (*arrow*). The nerve roots adhere to the walls of the thecal sac, particularly close to the diverticula.

### Suggested Reading

Charlesworth CH, Savy LE, Stevens J, Twomey B, Mitchell R. MRI demonstration of arachnoiditis in cauda equina syndrome of ankylosing spondylitis. *Neuroradiology* 1996;38:462.

# Spondylitis and Discitis, Pyogenic

## KEY FACTS

- Most instances of pyogenic spondylitis and discitis are caused by *Staphylococcus aureus* (60%), *Enterobacter* organisms (30%), *Escherichia coli, Pseudomonas* organisms, and *Klebsiella* organisms.
- Most instances arise from hematogenous dissemination (e.g., among drug users and immunodepressed patients), the ascending route (genitourinary tract manipulation), and direct inoculation (traumatic injuries and after an operation).
- Among adults infection begins in the vertebral end plates; in children the infection begins in the disc.
- These conditions usually occur among men between the sixth and seventh decades of life; the presenting symptoms are nonspecific (e.g., fever, pain, and elevated erythrocyte sedimentation rate).
- Plain films are not sensitive and remain normal 7 to 10 days after the onset of symptoms.
- In approximately 25% of cases, multiple levels are involved.

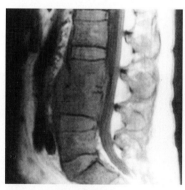

A

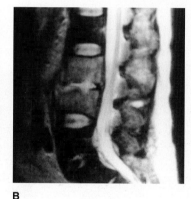

B

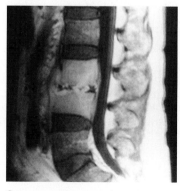

C

### FIGURE 24-2

**(A)** Midsagittal noncontrast T1-weighted MR image shows narrowing of L3-4 disc, erosion of the adjacent end plates, and anterior spinal and epidural soft-tissue abnormalities. **(B)** Corresponding T2-weighted image shows hyperintensity of the L3 and L4 vertebral bodies and disc. **(C)** After administration of contrast material, the vertebrae, disc, and epidural phlegmons become enhanced.

## Suggested Reading

Sklar EML, Post Donovan MJ, Lebwohl NH. Imaging of infections of the lumbosacral spine. *Neuroimaging Clin North Am* 1993;3:577.

# Epidural and Subdural Abscesses

### KEY FACTS

- Epidural and subdural abscesses occur secondary to extension of adjacent discitis or osteomyelitis (80%) or directly from hematogenous spread (common sources include the genitourinary tract, skin, and lungs).

- *Staphylococcus aureus* is the most common responsible organism.

- Abscesses are more common among middle-aged men.

- Symptoms are nonspecific, and they should be suspected when the following predisposing factors are present: diabetes, intravenous drug use, trauma, or immunocompromised state.

- In most instances, magnetic resonance (MR) images show enhancement of an extradural collection, which is related to the presence of phlegmon.

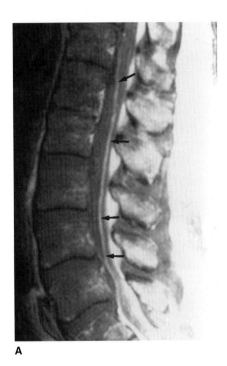

A

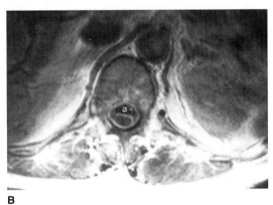

B

**FIGURE 24-3**    (A) Midsagittal postcontrast T1-weighted MR image shows an extensive epidural abscess (*arrows*) anteriorly. The dura marginating the posterior of the abscess is thick and enhanced. There is no osteomyelitis or discitis, suggesting a hematogenous origin of this abscess. (B) Axial postcontrast T1-weighted MR image of the same patient shows the ventral abscess (*a*).

## Suggested Reading

Numaguchi Y, Rigamonti D, Rothman MI, et al. Spinal epidural abscess: evaluation with gadolinium-enhanced MR imaging. *Radiographics* 1993;13:545.

# Tuberculosis

## KEY FACTS

- The incidence of tuberculosis is increasing because of immigration and acquired immunodeficiency syndrome (AIDS).
- The most common locations are the thoracic, lumbar, cervical, and sacral regions.
- Infection begins in the anteroinferior vertebral body and extends under ligaments skipping the discs; skip lesions are not uncommon.
- Tuberculosis occasionally involves the posterior elements.
- It is accompanied by considerable soft-tissue abnormality.
- Gibbus deformity is not an uncommon sequela.

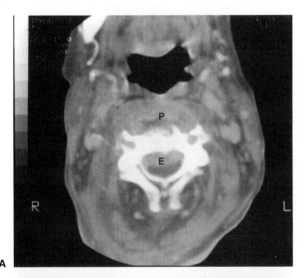

A

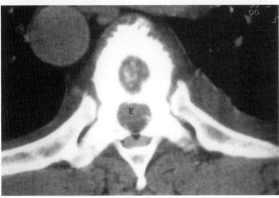

B

**FIGURE 24-4**

**(A)** Axial CT scan shows destruction of the anterior and interior aspect of C2 and a precervical (P) and ventral epidural (E) abscess. **(B)** Axial CT scan of a different patient shows destruction of the midbody of a thoracic vertebra. There is extension of the process into the ventral epidural space (E).

## Suggested Reading

Sharif HS, Morgan JL, al Shahed MS, al Thagafi MY. Role of CT and MR imaging in management of tuberculous spondylitis. *Radiol Clin North Am* 1995;33:787.

# *Guillain-Barré Syndrome*

## KEY FACTS

- Guillain-Barré syndrome is an inflammatory disorder that affects the peripheral nervous system.
- In 65% of instances it is preceded by a viral illness 3 to 6 weeks before the onset of neurologic symptoms.
- Most patients are younger than 18 years.
- The syndrome is pathologically characterized by demyelination and inflammation.
- It may extend into the spinal cord and present as transverse myelitis.

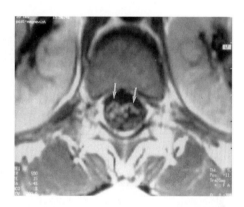

**FIGURE 24-5**
Axial postcontrast T1-weighted MR image shows enhancement and thickening of the ventral rootlets (*arrows*) of the cauda equina.

## Suggested Reading

Georgy BA, Chong B, Chamberlain M, Hesselink JR, Cheung G. MR of the spine in Guillain-Barre syndrome. *Am J Neuroradiol* 1994;15:300.

# *Hypertrophic Polyneuropathy*

## KEY FACTS

- The histologic features of hypertrophic polyneuropathy are demyelination and inflammation, which subside and lead to remyelination, producing the so-called onion bulb appearance of nerves.

- Common disorders included in this category are chronic primary inflammatory demyelinating polyneuropathy (probably the most common), Charcot-Marie-Tooth disease (also relatively common and occurring mostly among young women), and Dejerine-Sottas disease.

- Clinical symptoms include atrophy of the feet, legs, arms, and trunk, ataxia, and weakness.

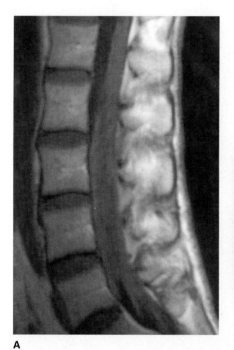

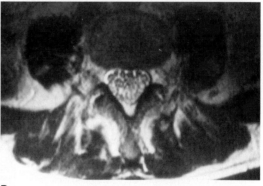

**A**    **B**

**FIGURE 24-6**    **(A)** Midsagittal postcontrast T1-weighted MR image shows diffuse thickening and enhancement of the cauda equina of a patient with Charcot-Marie-Tooth disease. **(B)** Axial T2-weighted MR image of the same patient shows hyperintense and thick lumbar nerve roots.

## Suggested Reading

Castillo M, Mukherji SK. MRI of enlarged dorsal ganglia, lumbar nerve roots, and cranial nerves in polyradiculoneuropathies. *Neuroradiology* 1996;38:516.

# *Rheumatoid Arthritis*

### KEY FACTS

- Rheumatoid arthritis occurs mostly among women 25 to 55 years of age.
- The disease affects the cervical region in 50% to 90% of patients and leads to C1-2 instability among 25% of them (this involvement carries a poor prognosis because it may result in spinal cord compression and sudden death).
- Pannus surrounding and eroding the dens occurs among 14% to 35% of patients.
- Other symptoms are basilar invagination, paresthesia, paresis, and muscle atrophy.

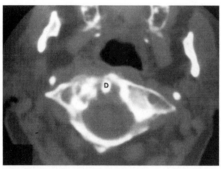

**A**

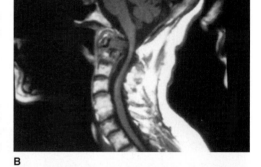

**B**

**FIGURE 24-7**

**(A)** Axial CT scan shows marked erosion of the dens (*D*) and anterior arch of C1. **(B)** Midsagittal T1-weighted MR image of a different patient shows destruction of the dens by pannus and compression of the cervicomedullary junction. **(C)** Corresponding T2-weighted image of the same patient as in **B** shows the pannus to be bright. The small area of hyperintensity (*arrow*) in the spinal cord is probably myelomalacia.

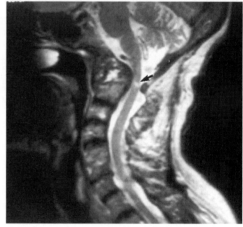

**C**

### Suggested Reading

Ruiz A, Post JD, Ganz WI. Inflammatory and infectious processes of the cervical spine. *Neuroimaging Clin North Am* 1995;5:401.

# 25   Trauma

## *Occipito-atlanto Dislocation*

### KEY FACTS

- Occipito-atlanto dislocation is an almost uniformly fatal injury caused by rupture of craniocervical ligaments (tectorial membrane, cruciate, apical, and alar ligaments) as the result of rapid deceleration with hyperflexion or hyperextension of the head.
- The injury is more common among children because of the large size of their heads.
- Normal basion (anterior lip foramen magnum) to dens distance should not exceed 12 mm for children or adults.
- A ratio (BC:OA) of the distance between basion (B) and posterior arch of C1 (C) divided by the distance between the anterior arch of C1 (A) and the opisthion (O) helps to establish anterior or posterior displacements in occipito-atlanto dislocations. A ratio greater than 1 is indicative of anterior displacement (note that it is difficult to reliably visualize the opisthion in more than 70% of lateral cervical spine radiographs).

*(continued)*

## *Occipito-atlanto Dislocation* (Continued)

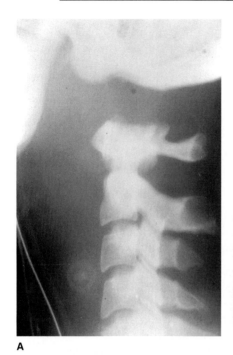

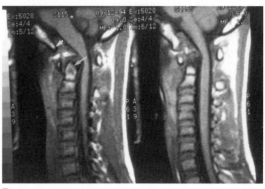

A                                          B

FIGURE 25-1    (A) Lateral radiograph shows separation of the occipital bone from the
atlas. (B) Sagittal T1-weighted MR images of a different patient shows
increased distance between the dens (*long arrow*) and the clivus (*short
arrow*). The dens is displaced posteriorly, and there is precervical
swelling. The cervicomedullary junction is compressed.

### Suggested Readings

Harris JH, Carson GC, Wagner LK. Radiologic diagnosis of traumatic occipitovertebral dis-
    sociation, I: normal occipitovertebral relationships on lateral radiographs of supine sub-
    jects. *Am J Roentgenol* 1994;162:881.
Harris JH, Carson GC, Wagner LK: Radiologic diagnosis of traumatic occipitovertebral dis-
    sociation, II: Comparison of three methods of detecting occipitovertebral relationships on
    lateral radiographs of supine subjects. *Am J Roentgenol* 1994;162:887.

# Jefferson Fracture

## KEY FACTS

- Jefferson fracture is the most common fracture of C1; it is caused by axial compression.
- This fracture generally results in bilateral fractures of the anterior and posterior arches but may be unilateral if the head is tilted on impact.
- Generally there is no spinal cord damage because the canal diameter is not greatly compromised.
- Vertebral arteries may be injured.
- The fracture is unstable if lateral masses of C1 are separated from the dens by more than 7 mm (implies torn transverse ligament).

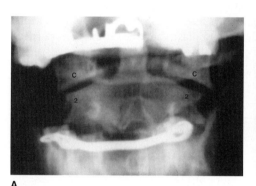 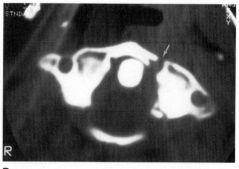

A                                              B

FIGURE 25-2    (A) Frontal open mouth shows outward displacement of the lateral masses (*C*) of C1 with respect to C2 (*2*). (B) Axial CT scan of a different patient shows a fracture (*arrow*) through the left anterior arch of C1.

## Suggested Reading

West OC, Anbari MM, Pilgram TK, Wilson AJ. Acute cervical spine trauma: diagnostic performance of single-view versus three-view radiographic screening. *Radiology* 1997;204:819.

# *Odontoid Fracture*

### KEY FACTS

- Odontoid fracture is the most common fracture of C2.
- *Type 1* occurs through the tip of the dens, is the least common type, and is stable; it may be confused with an os odontoideum.
- *Type 2* is the most common type and involves the base of the dens; it may be missed on axial computed tomographic (CT) scans. Plain radiographs and sagittal or coronal CT reformations are mandatory. Among adults this fracture disrupts the blood supply, and there is a high incidence of nonunion.
- *Type 3* extends from the base of the dens to the body of C2; if it extends into articular facets, the prognosis worsens.
- Os odontoideum is lack of assimilation of an occipital vertebra or a hypertrophied ossiculum terminale. It is always accompanied by hypoplasia of the remaining dens and may have hypoplastic anterior or posterior arches of C1 and instability of C1-2.
- Vertical fractures are a newly recognized and rare type of injury to the dens.

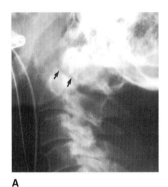 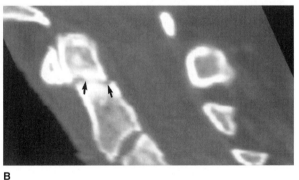

A        B

**FIGURE 25-3**    **(A)** Lateral radiograph shows type 2 fracture (*arrows*) of the dens. **(B)** Sagittal CT reformation of a different patient shows type 2 dens fracture (*arrows*).

### Suggested Reading
Castillo M, Mukherji SK. Vertical fractures of the dens. *Am J Neuroradiol* 1996;17:1627.

# *Hangman's Fracture*

**KEY FACTS**

- Hangman's fracture of both C2 pedicles is secondary to hyperextension, compression, and distraction, which may produce instant death due to spinal cord transection.

- Avulsion of the anterior aspect of the end plates of C2 and C3 may be present.

- Pedicle fractures are usually bilateral, but asymmetric fractures may extend to the lamina, facets, or vertebral body.

- Associated disk herniations may occur.

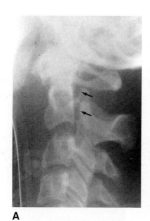
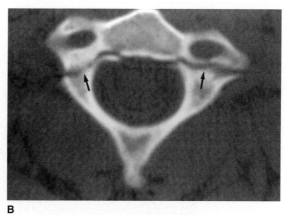

A    B

**F I G U R E  2 5 - 4**    **(A)** Lateral radiograph shows fractures (*arrows*) of the pars interarticularis of C2. **(B)** Axial CT scan of a different patient shows fractures (*arrows*) through the pars interarticularis.

## Suggested Reading

Mirvis SE, Young JWR, Lim C, Greenberg J. Hangman's fracture: radiologic assessment in 27 cases. *Radiology* 1987;163:713.

# *Atlantodental Instability*

---

## KEY FACTS

- Atlantodental instability is related to laxity or rupture of the transverse ligament.
- A normal atlantodental space measures 2 to 3 mm in adults and may be as wide as 5 mm in young children.
- The most common causes of atlantodental instability include trauma, pharyngitis and tonsillitis (especially among children), rheumatoid arthritis, ankylosing spondylitis, Down syndrome, and os odontoideum.
- The best diagnostic modality for assessing stability is fluoroscopy and plain radiography.

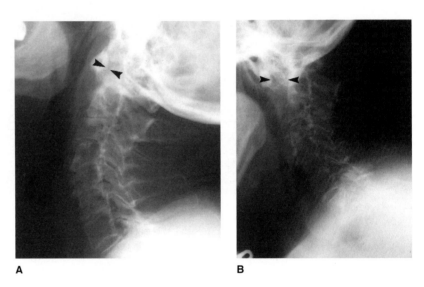

A                                                    B

FIGURE 25-5   (A) Extension lateral radiograph of a patient with rheumatoid arthritis shows a normal atlantodental space (*arrowheads*). (B) On the flexion view, there is considerable widening of the atlantodental space (*arrowheads*).

## Suggested Reading

Smoker WRK. Craniovertebral junction: normal anatomy, craniometry, and congenital abnormalities. *Radiographics* 1994;14:255.

# *Facet Dislocation*

## KEY FACTS

- Facet dislocation is an injury produced by a combination of flexion and rotation, which leads to tearing of the articular capsule and sliding of the superior facet forward on inferior facet.

- In unilateral subluxation and dislocation, the respective vertebral body rotates and slides anteriorly (<50%) on the vertebra below.

- An even greater force tears both articular capsules and produces bilateral facet dislocations, which result in >50% anterior displacement of the respective vertebral body on the vertebra below, producing a very unstable injury (delayed instability is also very common).

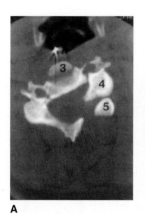

**A**

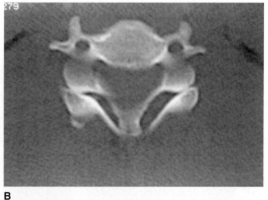

**B**

**FIGURE 25-6**
**(A)** Axial CT scan of a patient with left facetal dislocation shows posterior luxated superior articular process of C5 (*5*) and anterior location of the inferior articular process of C4 (*4*). A portion of the C3 vertebral body (*3*) is present anteriorly. **(B)** Axial CT scan of a different patient shows bilateral facetal dislocations. **(C)** Midsagittal T2-weighted MR image of the same patient as in **B** shows anterior subluxation of C5 on C6, disc herniation at this level, disruption of the anterior and posterior longitudinal ligaments, prevertebral edema, and spinal cord hyperintensity.

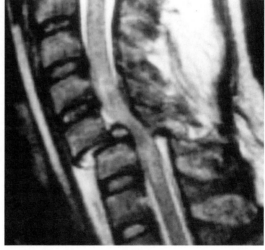

**C**

## Suggested Reading

Yetkin Z, Osborn AG, Giles DS, Haughton VM. Uncovertebral and facet joint dislocations in cervical articular pillar fractures: CT evaluation. *Am J Neuroradiol* 1985;6:633.

# Vertebral Body Compression Fracture, Cervical and Thoracic Spine

## KEY FACTS

- Vertebral body compression fracture is the most common type of injury to the cervical and thoracic spine. It is caused by flexion and axial loading.
- The fracture may be unstable. Depending on the degree of flexion, there may be tearing of interspinous, capsular, or posterior longitudinal ligaments. The disc may rupture, and anterior subluxation of the involved vertebra may occur.
- CT scans show bone fragments that may be displaced into the spinal canal and unsuspected fractures of the posterior elements (bursting of a vertebral body may occur).
- The most severe flexion fracture in the cervical region is the teardrop type, in which a posterior bone fragment is displaced, damaging the spinal cord.

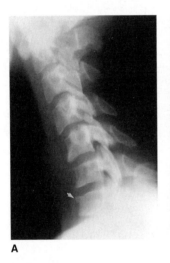 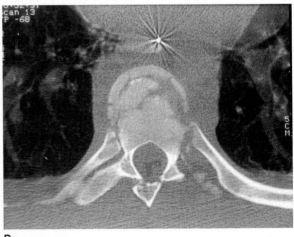

A                                             B

FIGURE 25-7    (A) Lateral radiograph shows flexion injury that resulted in compression of the C7 vertebral body, superior end plate, and chip fracture (*arrow*) of the anterosuperior body. There is kyphotic angulation of the cervical spine, implying a ligamentous injury. **(B)** Axial CT scan of a different patient shows compression of the mid-to-anterior aspects of the body of a midthoracic vertebral body.

## Suggested Reading

Berquist TH. Imaging of adult cervical spine trauma. *Radiographics* 1988;8:667.

# Compression Fracture, Lumbar Spine

## KEY FACTS

- Compression fractures of the lumbar spine result from axial loading or exaggerated flexion of the lumbar spine.

- These fractures produce loss of height of the vertebral body and if severe enough may displace bone fragments into the spinal canal.

- If the compression involves only the anterior third of a vertebra, the ligaments are generally intact, and the injury is considered stable.

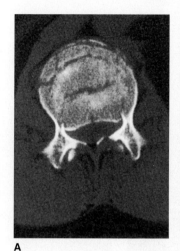 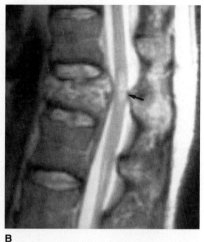

A                                    B

**FIGURE 25-8**        **(A)** Axial CT scan shows compression fracture of L1 with displacement of the posterior cortex into the spinal canal. **(B)** Midsagittal T2-weighted MR image of a different patient shows compression of L1 with narrowing of the spinal canal. The high signal intensity in the spinal cord (*arrow*) represents edema. The involved vertebral body is bright because of a combination of edema and hemorrhage.

## Suggested Reading

Saifudding A, Noordeen H, Taylor BA, Bayley I. The role of imaging in the diagnosis of thoracolumbar burst fractures: current concepts and a review of the literature. *Skeletal Radiol* 1996;25:603.

# Chance-Type Fracture

### KEY FACTS

- Chance-type fractures are injuries produced by hyperflexion associated with falls or vehicular accidents while wearing only a lap seatbelt.

- With Chance fractures, there is disruption of the posterior ligament complex with shearing of pedicles and vertebral body; occasionally a Chance fracture occurs through the disc, and all Chance fractures may be associated with injuries to the abdominal organs.

- Severe disruption of facet joints leads to complete dislocation and produces a naked facet sign on CT scans.

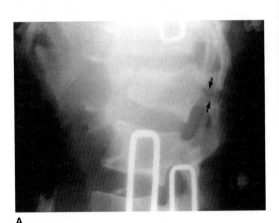

A

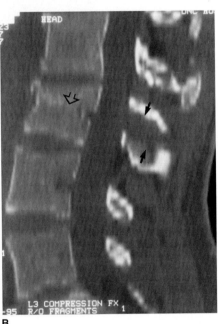

B

**FIGURE 25-9**    (A) Lateral radiograph shows fracture (*arrows*) through the posterior elements of L1 and compression of the vertebral body. (B) Sagittal CT reformation of a different patient shows fracture involving the posterior elements (*solid arrows*) and midbody (*open arrow*) of L3. L3 is slightly wedged, and its anterior cortex is buckled inward.

### Suggested Reading

Terk MR, Hume-Neal M, Fraipont M, Ahmadi J, Colletti PM. Injury to the posterior ligament complex in patients with acute spinal trauma: evaluation by MR imaging. *Am J Roentgenol* 1997;168:1481.

# Spinal Cord Contusion

## KEY FACTS

- Bone injury does not accurately correlate with neurologic findings in more than 65% of instances of spinal trauma, especially among children.

- Hemorrhagic contusions are seen as central areas of hypointensity (deoxyhemoglobin) surrounded by edema on T2-weighted magnetic resonance (MR) images and have a poor prognosis with little likelihood of recovery.

- Nonhemorrhagic contusions produce edema, have normal T1-weighted MR images and areas of hyperintensity on T2-weighted MR images, and have a moderately good prognosis.

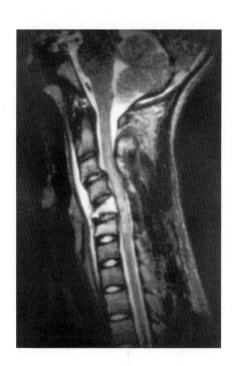

**FIGURE 25-10**
Midsagittal T2-weighted MR image of a patient with compression fractures of C5 and C6 shows high signal intensity in the spinal cord at that level compatible with edema.

## Suggested Reading
Davis PC, Reisner A, Hudgins PA, Davis WE, O'Brien MS. Spinal injuries in children: role of MR. *Am J Neuroradiol* 1993;14:607.

# Acute Traumatic Spinal Cord Hematoma and Transection

## KEY FACTS

- A large number of patients with spinal cord hematoma have neurologic deficits with no plain radiographic correlation.
- Magnetic resonance imaging (MRI) reveals three patterns of spinal cord injury, as follows:
- *Type 1:* initial central hypointensity on T1-weighted MR images evolving to hyperintensity, probably related to hemorrhage (deoxyhemoglobin); correlates with the highest degree of severity; usually there is no neurologic improvement (Kulkarni type 1).
- *Type 2:* initial cord hyperintensity on T2-weighted MR images resolving rapidly (3 to 7 days); most likely related to edema; patients improve considerably (Kulkarni type 2).
- *Type 3:* mixed lesions including early small central area of hypointensity in the spinal cord surrounded by edema with eventual partial resolution of MR findings and some clinical improvement (Kulkarni type 3).
- In instances of spinal cord transection there is complete pulping of the cord or total disruption; all neurologic deficits are permanent.
- Although the presence of spinal cord intramedullary lesions detected at MRI have prognostic implications for the patient, surgical treatment usually is provided in the acute setting only for extramedullary abnormalities (hematoma, retropulsed bone fragments, and disc herniation) that compress the spinal cord.

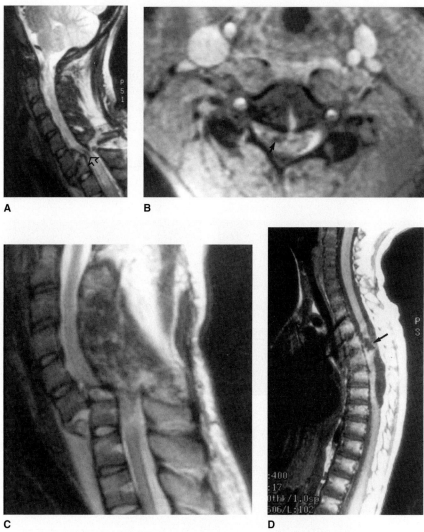

**A**   **B**

**C**   **D**

**FIGURE 25-11**   (A) Midsagittal T2-weighted MR image of a patient with bilateral facet dislocation at C6 and C7 shows low signal intensity (*arrow*) inside the spinal cord compatible with hematoma. (B) Axial gradient echo (T2*)–weighted image of a different patient with a cervical compression fracture shows low signal intensity (*arrow*) inside the spinal cord suggesting hematoma. (C) Midsagittal T2-weighted MR image shows fracture dislocation of C6-7 with spinal cord transection. (D) Midsagittal T1-weighted MR image of a child without abnormalities shows transection (*arrow*) of upper thoracic spinal cord.

## Suggested Reading

Quencer RM, Nunez D, Green BA. Controversies in imaging acute cervical spine trauma. *Am J Neuroradiol* 1997;18:1866.

# Nerve Root Avulsion

### KEY FACTS

- Nerve root avulsion generally is caused by traction injury to the extremities (in the lower cervical spine, they are related to traction of the arms; in the lower spine, they are related to lumbosacral spinal or pelvic fractures).

- With complete avulsion, the nerve roots retract, leaving behind fluid-filled pseudomeningoceles.

- Penetration of the meninges by bone fragments, bullets, or stab wounds may cause dural tears.

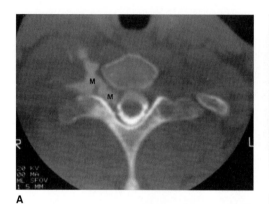 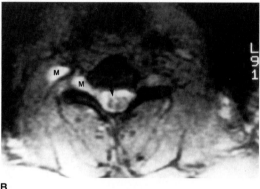

A                                                B

**FIGURE 25-12**    **(A)** Axial postmyelographic CT scan shows contrast-filled pseudomeningocele (*M*) caused by avulsion of nerve root and its sleeve and extravasation of contrast medium. **(B)** Axial T2-weighted MR image of a different patient shows high signal intensity from pseudomeningocele (*M*) and fissure (*arrow*) in the spinal cord.

### Suggested Reading

Mukherji SK, Castillo M, Wagle AG. The brachial plexus. *Semin Ultrasound CT MRI* 1996;17:519.

# 26   Congenital Anomalies

## *Myelocele and Myelomeningocele*

**KEY FACTS**

- Myelocele and myelomeningocele are midline bone defects through which meninges or neural placode (unfolded spinal cord) are visible.
- In a myelomeningocele (the most common type, 0.1% of live births), the neural placode and meninges protrude above the skin; it almost always occurs in the context of a Chiari II malformation and is generally sporadic but may affect subsequent siblings.
- In a myelocele (less common), the neural placode is flush with the skin.
- Both entities are untethered and closed at birth; imaging is performed for recurrent symptoms.
- For practical purposes all spinal cords retether (because of scar), and imaging studies are used to exclude other abnormalities, such as syringomyelia (30% to 75%), diastematomyelia (30%), lipoma, dermoid, and epidermoid.

*(continued)*

# *Myelocele and Myelomeningocele* *(Continued)*

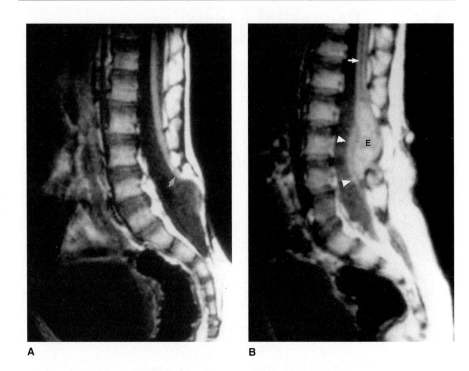

A                                    B

FIGURE 26-1    **(A)** Midsagittal T1-weighted MR image of a patient with a repaired myelocele and symptoms of retethering. The cord (*arrow*) terminates at the level of the dysraphism. **(B)** Midsagittal T1-weighted MR image of a different patient after repair of a myelomeningocele shows low position of spinal cord (*arrowheads*). The cord drapes over an epidermoid (*E*). Note cyst (*arrow*) within distal spinal cord.

## Suggested Reading

Armstrong DC. Congenital malformations of the spine. *Top Magn Reson Imaging* 1993;5:131.

# *Lipomyelocele and Lipomyelomeningocele*

### KEY FACTS

- Lipomyelocele and lipomyelomeningocele are midline bony defects of the spine covered by skin that may have a dermal sinus, hairy patch, or hemangioma above the intergluteal fold.

- In a lipomyelocele, meninges and neural placode are located at the level of a spina bifida lesion but covered by a lipoma and skin.

- In a lipomyelomeningocele, the meninges and neural placode protrude through a bone opening but are covered by a lipoma and skin; this lipoma is in direct contact with the surface of the neural placode, and patients have a prominent mass in the low back.

- Intraspinal lipoma (generally lumbosacral) is a collection of intradural fat contiguous with the dorsal surface of the tethered spinal cord.

- Other entities that can be considered occult dysraphism include anterior sacral and intrasacral meningocele and diastematomyelia.

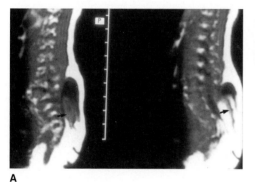 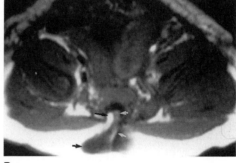

A                                    B

**FIGURE 26-2**     **(A)** Parasagittal T1-weighted MR images of a patient with a lipomyelomeningocele shows fluid-filled protrusion containing tethered spinal cord (*arrows*). The dysraphism is covered by fat (which continues into the level of the placode) and is covered by skin. **(B)** Axial T1-weighted MR image of the same patient shows continuation of the fat (*long black arrow*) into the spinal canal and in immediate vicinity of an unfolded and low positioned spinal cord (*white arrows*). Note fluid-filled protrusion (*short black arrow*) into the subcutaneous tissues.

### Suggested Reading

Scatliff JH, Kendall BE, Kingsley DP, Britton J, Gran DN, Hayward RD. Closed spinal dysraphism: analysis of clinical, radiological, and surgical findings in 104 consecutive patients. *Am J Roentgenol* 1989;152:1049.

# *Lipoma*

KEY FACTS

- Filar lipoma is the most common intraspinal lipoma. It occurs among 1% to 6% of the population and is generally an incidental and asymptomatic finding.
- The filum terminale is thickened (generally its normal size should not exceed that of neighboring nerve roots) and has fat within it.
- In the presence of filar lipoma, if the conus medullaris is normal in position, the findings are probably not clinically significant; however, if the conus medullaris is abnormally low, consider the diagnosis of tight filum terminale syndrome.
- Intradural lipomas are rare and are found more often in the cervical region. Most become symptomatic by 5 years of age and result in paresis, spasticity, sensory loss, weakness, and bowel or bladder dysfunction.

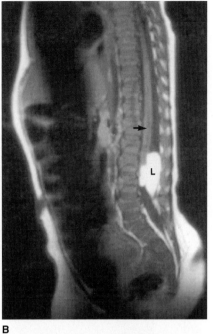

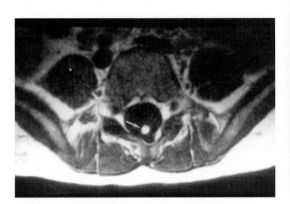

**A**

**B**

**FIGURE 26-3**

**(A)** Axial T1-weighted MR image shows lipoma (*arrow*) in a thick filum terminale in a patient with a tight filum terminale syndrome. **(B)** Midsagittal T1-weighted MR image shows intraspinal lipoma (*L*), low positioned spinal cord at the L3 level, and a possible spinal cord cyst (*arrow*). **(C)** Midsagittal T1-weighted MR image of a different patient shows a lipoma (*L*) in an expanded cervical spinal canal.

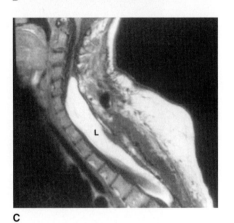

**C**

### Suggested Reading

Altman NR, Altman DH. MR imaging of spinal dysraphism. *Am J Neuroradiol* 1987;8:533.

# Dermoid and Epidermoid

## KEY FACTS

- Dermoid and epidermoid lesions account for 3% to 17% of all spinal tumors among children; 20% to 30% are associated with a dermal sinus tract.

- The histologic features of epidermoid are a fibrous capsule and squamous epithelium; dermoid contains skin appendages (hair follicles and sebaceous and sweat glands).

- Chemical meningitis occurs after rupture of dermoid and epidermoid tumors.

- The most common location is the lumbosacral spine.

- Epidermoids contain liquid cholesterol and are difficult to visualize at magnetic resonance imaging (MRI). Dermoids contain solid cholesterol and have signal intensities similar to those of fat.

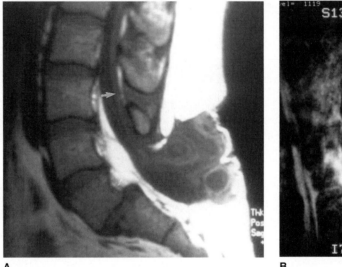 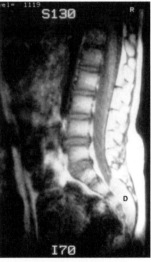

A                                           B

**FIGURE 26-4**    **(A)** Midsagittal T1-weighted MR image shows a mass in the subcutaneous lumbar region. This epidermoid is mostly isointense to cerebrospinal fluid but also contains some serpiginous areas of intermediate signal intensity. The spinal cord (*arrow*) is dysplastic and tethered inferiorly by the lesion. **(B)** Midsagittal T1-weighted MR image of a different patient shows hyperintense dermoid (*D*) in the distal spinal canal.

## Suggested Reading

Roeder MB, Bazan C, Jinkins JR. Ruptured spinal dermoid cyst with chemical arachnoiditis and disseminated intracranial lipid droplets. *Neuroradiology* 1995;37:146.

# Diastematomyelia

## KEY FACTS

- Diastematomyelia is sagittal splitting of the spinal cord by a bony or fibrous band, which usually originates from posterior elements and courses ventrally to join the vertebral body.

- This condition occurs among 5% of persons with scoliosis and approximately 30% of patients with myelomeningocele.

- About 50% of instances of diastematomyelia occur in the thoracic spine and 50% in lumbar region.

- About 50% of hemicords lie in a single dural sheath, and 50% of hemicords are enveloped by individual dural sheaths.

- Vertebral body abnormalities and overlying skin lesions occur among most patients.

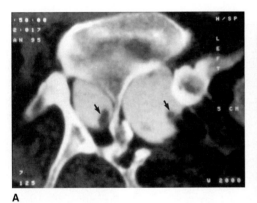

**A**

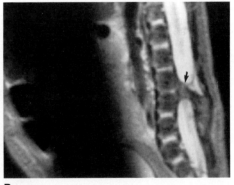

**B**

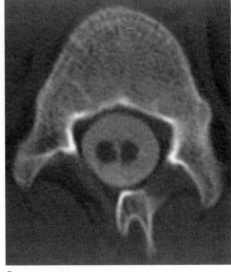

**C**

## FIGURE 26-5

**(A)** Axial postmyelographic CT scan shows bone spur dividing the spinal canal and each half containing a hemicord (*arrows*). The neural arch is dysplastic. **(B)** Midsagittal T2-weighted MR image of a different patient shows bone spur (*arrow*) traversing the spinal canal. **(C)** Axial postmyelographic CT scan of a patient with internal diastematomyelia shows one thecal sac, two hemicords, and no spur.

## Suggested Reading

Anderson NG, Jorda S, MacFarlane MR, Lovell-Smith M. Diastematomyelia: diagnosis by prenatal sonography. *Am J Roentgenol* 1994;163:911.

# Caudal Regression Syndrome

## KEY FACTS

- Caudal regression syndrome is a rare and complex anomaly that includes absence of the lower vertebrae, anal atresia, malformed genitalia, renal abnormalities, and rarely fusion of the lower extremities (sirenomyelia).
- About 16% of patients are the offspring of women with diabetes.
- Most patients have a neurogenic bladder, motor weakness, and foot deformities.
- In one type, the sacrum is absent and the distal conus (wedge-shaped) and cauda equina are not completely formed. In a different type the spinal cord is dysplastic and tethered at the level of agenesis.
- Associated abnormalities are diastematomyelia, intraspinal lipoma, dermoid, and dermal sinuses.

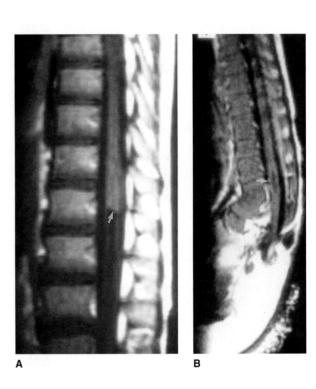

**FIGURE 26-6**
(A) Midsagittal T1-weighted MR image of a patient with partial sacral agenesis shows truncated conus medullaris (*arrow*) and a sparse cauda equina. (B) Image of a different patient with absence of the sacrum and distal lumbar spine. Spinal cord is tethered at the level of the agenesis and contains a small cyst (*arrow*).

A                    B

## Suggested Reading

Nievelstein RA, Valk J, Smit LM, Vermeij-Keers C. MR of the caudal regression syndrome: embryologic implications. *Am J Neuroradiol* 1994;15:1021.

# *HEAD AND NECK*

# 27  Neck Masses

## *Nasopharyngeal Space Masses*

### KEY FACTS

- The most common tumors in the nasopharyngeal space include squamous cell carcinoma (>80%), adenocarcinoma, minor salivary gland tumors, and lymphoma.
- It is not clear whether tobacco and alcohol use are significant risk factors.
- Nasopharyngeal squamous cell carcinoma is more common in men older than 60 years of age and of Chinese origin.
- Common symptoms include adenopathy (>50%), serous otitis media (caused by obstruction of Eustachian tube orifice), nasal obstruction, epistaxis, and neurologic dysfunction caused by invasion of the base of the skull or cavernous sinus.
- Tumors begin in the fossa of Rosenmüller and have local extension with initial metastases to the lateral retropharyngeal nodes of Rouviere, spinal accessory (level 5) nodes, and last to the internal jugular nodes (level 2, 3, and 4).
- Nodes are present in 50% of patients at diagnosis and decrease survival time by half.
- Both computed tomography (CT) and magnetic resonance imaging (MRI) are poor in the detection of recurrences.

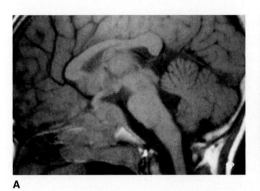
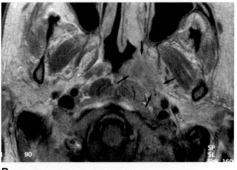

A                                          B

**FIGURE 27-1** (A) Midsagittal noncontrast T1-weighted MR image shows carcinoma from nasopharynx extending into the sphenoid sinus and destroying the sella and clivus. (B) Postcontrast T1-weighted MR image of a patient with early cancer shows lesion (*arrows*) in region of the left fossa of Rosenmüller.

## Suggested Reading
Xhong VFH, Fan YF. Detection of recurrent nasopharyngeal carcinoma: MR imaging versus CT. *Radiology* 1997;202:463.

# *Parapharyngeal Space Masses*

### KEY FACTS

- A normal parapharyngeal space contains fat, the third division of the trigeminal nerves, branches of the internal maxillary artery, and the ascending pharyngeal artery and veins.

- The parapharyngeal space is divided into a prestyloid compartment (80% of masses occur here and are mostly pleomorphic adenomas) and a poststyloid compartment (20% of masses arise here and are mostly neurogenic tumors and paragangliomas).

- In examinations of children, consider second branchial cleft cysts and abscesses.

- Squamous cell carcinoma usually arises from the adjacent pharyngeal mucosal space and invades the parapharyngeal space secondarily.

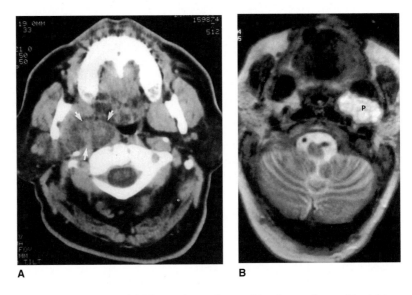

A                                         B

FIGURE 27-2        (A) Axial CT scan shows pleomorphic adenoma (*arrows*) in right parapharyngeal space. (B) Axial T2-weighted MR image of a different patient shows bright pleomorphic adenoma (*P*) in the left parapharyngeal space.

### Suggested Reading

Vogl TJ, Balzer JO. Base of skull, nasopharynx, and parapharyngeal space. *Neuroimaging Clin North Am* 1996;6:357.

# *Parotid Space Masses*

## KEY FACTS

- A normal parotid space contains the parotid gland, nodes, retromandibular vein (which arbitrarily divides the gland into deep and superficial portions on images), facial nerve (which anatomically divides the gland into deep and superficial portions), and external carotid artery.

- For a child with a parotid mass, consider hemangioma, lymphangioma, and first branchial cleft cyst.

- For patients with acquired immunodeficiency syndrome (AIDS) who have parotid masses, consider benign lymphoepithelial cysts, infection, and lymphoma.

- The most common tumors in the parotid space are benign mixed tumor (pleomorphic adenoma) (>80%), Warthin's tumor (especially among older men with bilateral parotid masses), mucoepidermoid carcinoma, adenoid cystic carcinoma (especially with multiple cranial nerve deficits caused by perineural tumor spread), metastases, and lymphoma (especially for patients with multiple masses).

- Facial nerve palsy in the presence of a parotid mass implies malignant growth and a poor prognosis.

- MRI reveals that benign tumors are hyperintense on T2-weighted images and malignant tumors are hypointense on T2-weighted images.

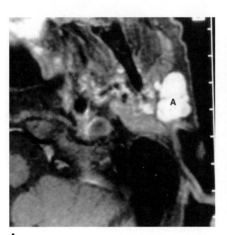
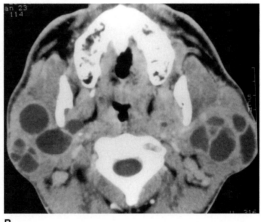

A       B

**FIGURE 27-3**      **(A)** Axial postcontrast fat-suppressed T1-weighted MR image shows enhancing pleomorphic adenoma (*A*) in the left parotid gland. **(B)** Axial CT scan of a patient with AIDS shows multiple lymphoepithelial cysts in the parotid glands.

## Suggested Reading

Som PM, Biller HF. High-grade malignancies of the parotid gland: identification with MR imaging. *Radiology* 1989;173:823.

# Retropharyngeal Space Masses

### KEY FACTS

- The retropharyngeal compartment is a potential space that contains fat and medial and lateral retropharyngeal nodes (between the prevertebral muscles and pharyngeal constrictor muscles) and extends from the base of the skull to T3.
- The most common lesions of this space are inflammatory processes (especially among children), which include reactive adenopathy and abscesses.
- Among adults, adenopathy at this level suggests metastatic disease until proved otherwise.
- Other lesions that involve the retropharyngeal space include hemangioma, lipoma, lymphoma, and direct invasion by squamous cell carcinoma.

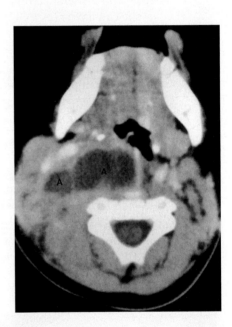

**FIGURE 27-4**
Axial postcontrast CT scan shows septated retropharyngeal abscess (*A*).

## Suggested Reading

Davis WL, Harnsberger HR, Smoker WRK, et al. Retropharyngeal space: evaluation of normal anatomy and disease with CT and MR imaging. *Radiology* 1990;174:59.

# *Oropharyngeal Space Masses*

## KEY FACTS

- Only 7% of masses in the oropharyngeal space are malignant, but more than 90% of malignant lesions are squamous cell carcinoma, followed by lymphoma, adenoid cystic carcinoma, mucoepidermoid carcinoma, and adenocarcinoma.

- Among children, the most common lesions at this location are hemangioma, lymphangioma or cystic hygroma, and tonsillar abscesses.

- Common risk factors for adults include tobacco and alcohol use and human immunodeficiency virus (HIV) infection.

- Most masses in the oropharyngeal space are found incidentally during routine physical examinations, but pain in the external auditory canal is an important clinical symptom.

- Most tumors in this region arise in the floor of the mouth (divided by mylohyoid muscle into submandibular [below] and sublingual [above] spaces), gingival folds, retromolar trigone, base of the tongue, and palate.

- Epidermoids and dermoids are distinct slow-growing lesions of the sublingual space that have a fatty appearance and may be identical to lipoma.

- Lingual thyroid should be included in the differential diagnosis of masses in the base of the tongue that enhance.

- Ranulas are retention cysts of salivary glands that may remain confined to the sublingual space (simple) or cross the mylohyoid muscle (diving); diving ranulas have no true walls.

*(continued)*

## *Oropharyngeal Space Masses (Continued)*

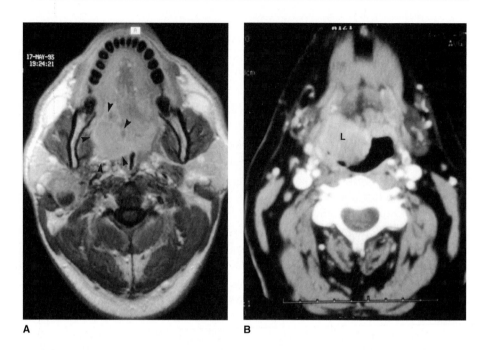

A                                              B

**FIGURE 27-5**    **(A)** Axial postcontrast T1-weighted MR image shows infiltrating carcinoma (*arrows*) at base of tongue. There is questionable extension across the midline. **(B)** Axial postcontrast CT scan shows enhancing lymphoma (*L*) in the right glossotonsillar region.

### Suggested Reading

Sigal R, Zagdanski AM, Schwaab G, et al. CT and MR imaging of squamous cell carcinoma of the tongue and floor of the mouth. *Radiographics* 1996;16:787.

# *Masticator Space Masses*

## KEY FACTS

- The masticator space normally contains the vertical mandibular ramus, masseter, temporalis, medial pterygoid and lateral pterygoid muscles, branches of the third division of the trigeminal nerve, and the inferior alveolar artery and vein.

- The most common lesions occurring here include odontogenic infection (remember that infections may track superiorly under the temporalis muscle), primary or secondary bone tumors, neurogenic tumors, lymphoma, or invasion from squamous cell carcinoma originating in the retromolar triangle.

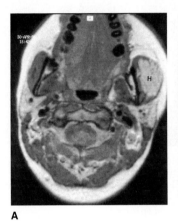 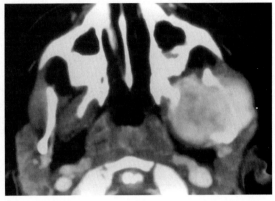

A                        B

**FIGURE 27-6**      **(A)** Axial noncontrast T1-weighted MR image shows bright hemangioma (*H*) in the left masseter muscle. **(B)** Axial postcontrast CT scan shows neurofibrosarcoma in the left masticator space. There is intense enhancement and destruction of the vertical mandibular ramus.

## Suggested Reading

Tryhus MR, Smoker WRK, Harnsberger HR. The normal and diseased masticator space. *Semin Ultrasound CT MR* 1990;11:476.

# Buccal Space Masses

## KEY FACTS

- The buccal space is posterolateral to the lower maxilla and contains mostly fat but also carries the facial artery and vein and distal parotid duct; its lateral margin is the buccinator muscle.

- The processes affecting this space are similar to those involving the masticator space and in most instances represent extension from a pathologic condition in the masticator space into the buccinator (buccal) space.

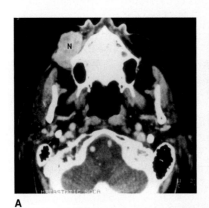 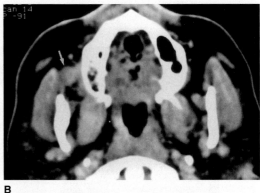

A          B

**FIGURE 27-7**      **(A)** Axial postcontrast CT scan shows nodal metastasis (*N*) from basal cell cancer. **(B)** Axial CT scan of a different patient shows buccal space pleomorphic adenoma (*arrow*).

## Suggested Reading

Tart RP, Kotzur IM, Mancuso AA, Glantz MS, Mukherji SK. CT and MR imaging of the buccal space and buccal space masses. *Radiographics* 1995;15:531.

# Sublingual and Submandibular Space Masses

KEY FACTS

- The sublingual space is superomedial to the mylohyoid muscle and mainly contains the tongue, lingual neurovascular plexus, sublingual glands and ducts, and Wharton's ducts.

- The most common pathologic conditions affecting the sublingual space are squamous cell carcinoma, tumors of the sublingual gland, cellulitis and abscesses, calculi, ranulas, lymphangioma, dermoid or epidermoid, ectopic thyroid, and hemangioma (among children).

- The submandibular space is inferolateral to the mylohyoid muscle, superior to the hyoid bone, and medial to the horizontal ramus of the mandible. It contains most of the submandibular gland, nodes, anterior belly of the digastric muscle, and facial vein and artery.

- Most common pathologic conditions affecting the submandibular space are metastases, invasion by squamous cell cancer from the mouth, submandibular gland tumors, lipoma, dermoid or epidermoid, ranula, infection, second branchial cleft cyst, and lymphangioma.

*(continued)*

# Sublingual and Submandibular Space Masses
## (Continued)

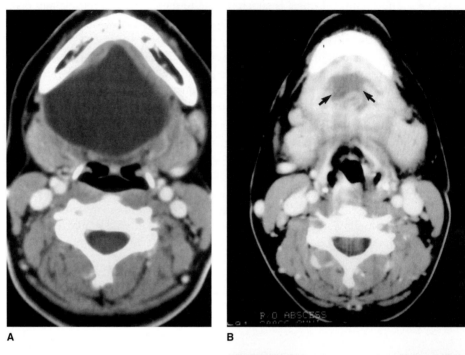

A

B

### FIGURE 27-8

(A) Axial postcontrast CT scan shows large dermoid in the sublingual space. (B) Axial postcontrast CT scan of a different patient shows necrotic abscess (*arrows*) in the sublingual space. (C) Axial postcontrast CT scan shows bilateral plunging ranulas (*R*) in the submandibular compartments.

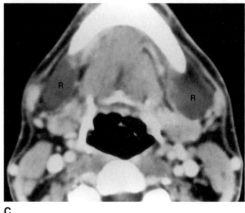

C

## Suggested Reading

Harnsberger HR. *Handbook of head and neck imaging.* 2nd ed. St. Louis: Mosby, 1995: 120–149.

# Carotid Space Masses

**KEY FACTS**

- The carotid space normally contains the internal carotid artery and its sheath; internal jugular vein; cranial nerves 9, 10, 11, and 12; nodes; and the sympathetic plexus.

- The most common lesions are carotid body tumor (paraganglioma arising at the common carotid artery bifurcation, 10% are multiple, 10% are malignant, and they occur in the fifth decade of life), schwannoma (usually from the vagus nerve), nodal metastases (from airway squamous cell carcinoma or lymphoma), and extracranial meningioma.

- Most lesions present as indolent masses in lateral neck.

- Vascular abnormalities such as ectatic arteries, pseudoaneurysm, and jugular vein thrombosis may affect this space.

- Remember the jugular veins are normally asymmetric in size.

*(continued)*

## *Carotid Space Masses* (Continued)

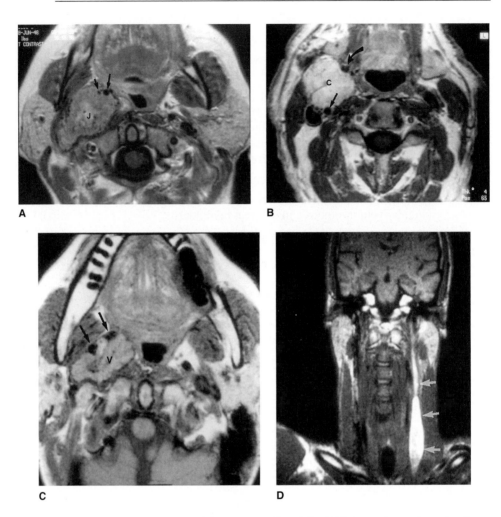

**FIGURE 27-9**    (A) Axial postcontrast T1-weighted MR image shows glomus jugulare (*j*) displacing the internal (*long arrow*) and external (*short arrow*) carotid arteries anteriorly. (B) Axial postcontrast T1-weighted MR image shows carotid body tumor (*c*) splaying the external (*curved arrow*) and internal (*straight arrow*) carotid arteries. (C) Axial postcontrast T1-weighted MR image shows anterior displacement of internal and external carotid arteries (*arrows*) by glomus vagale tumor (*V*). (D) Coronal noncontrast T1-weighted MR image shows hyperintense thrombus (*arrows*) occluding left internal jugular vein.

### Suggested Reading
Chong VF, Fan YF. Pictorial review: radiology of the carotid space. *Clin Radiol* 1996;51:762.

# *Laryngeal Masses*

### KEY FACTS

- The larynx extends from the valleculae to the space between the cricoid and first tracheal ring; the supraglottis begins with the tip of the epiglottis and ends in the laryngeal ventricle; the glottis is the true vocal cords; the infraglottis extends from the undersurface of the true vocal cords to the bottom of the cricoid.

- The most common pathologic conditions include squamous cell carcinoma, laryngocele, thyroglossal duct cyst, stenosis, and trauma.

- Most supraglottic tumors are squamous cell carcinoma; if the tumor stops at the laryngeal ventricle, supraglottic laryngectomy is performed (best voice-saving procedure).

- If the tumor respects the anterior commissure and involves less than the anterior third of the contralateral true cord, vertical hemilaryngectomy may be performed (anterior commissure normally measures <1 mm in width).

- If the tumor has infraglottic extension (1 cm below laryngeal ventricle), total laryngectomy is needed.

- Report for all laryngeal tumors the following information: nodal stage, cartilage invasion (relative contraindication to radiation), and status of infraglottis and midline.

- MRI is better for depicting cartilage invasion, but overestimation may occur because this modality does not allow one to differentiate tumor from inflammation.

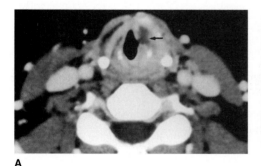
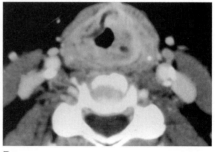

**A**                                           **B**

**FIGURE 27-10**      (A) Axial postcontrast CT scan shows carcinoma of the left true vocal cord. The laryngeal ventricle (*arrow*) is dilated and fluid filled. (B) Axial postcontrast CT scan of a different patient shows circumferential involvement by carcinoma of the true vocal cords.

### Suggested Reading

Becker M, Zbaren P, Laeng H, Stoupis C, Porcellini B, Vock P. Neoplastic invasion of the laryngeal cartilage: comparison of MR imaging and CT with histopathologic correlation. *Radiology* 1995;194:661.

# Nodal Metastases

KEY FACTS

- About 50% of all squamous cell carcinomas of the upper airway have nodal metastases at presentation; nodal metastases eventually develop in as many as 80% of these patients.
- The superior group of nodes is the lateral pharyngeal nodes (first order drainage of nasopharynx) and the jugulodigastric nodes.
- Below the jugulodigastric nodes, adenopathy may be classified as follows:
- *Level 1:* submandibular and submental nodes.
- *Level 2:* internal jugular chain above hyoid bone.
- *Level 3:* internal jugular chain between hyoid bone and cricoid cartilage.
- *Level 4:* internal jugular chain below cricoid cartilage.
- *Level 5:* spinal accessory chains.
- *Level 6:* nodes related to thyroid gland.
- *Level 7:* central compartment below the hyoid (tracheoesophageal and anterior cervical chain).
- Internal jugular nodes are the eventual drainage site for the entire neck; a size >15 mm diameter or central low density (necrosis) >3 mm diameter are compatible with metastases.
- The most common cause of nodal metastases is squamous cell carcinoma, lymphoma is the second most common (particularly Hodgkin's lymphoma) and results in moderately to enlarged nodes.
- The most common cause of completely cavitated nodes is papillary thyroid carcinoma (particularly at level 4).
- Differential diagnosis of calcified nodes includes tuberculosis, treated lymphoma, and metastases from neuroblastoma and papillary thyroid carcinoma.
- Differential diagnosis of hemorrhagic nodes includes metastases from renal cell, thyroid, and breast carcinoma.
- Nodes that are bright on precontrast T1-weighted MR images include those containing thyroglobulin and melanoma.

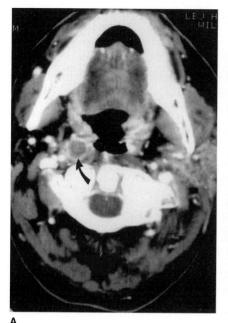

A

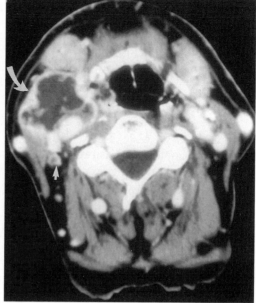

B

## FIGURE 27-11

(A) Axial postcontrast CT scan shows right-sided necrotic lateral retropharyngeal node of Rouviere (*arrow*). (B) Axial postcontrast CT scan of a different patient shows right level 1 (*curved arrow*) and level 5 (*short arrow*) necrotic nodes. (C) Axial postcontrast CT scan of a different patient shows level 1 (*short arrows*), level 2 (*long arrows*), and a left level 5 (*curved arrow*) necrotic nodes.

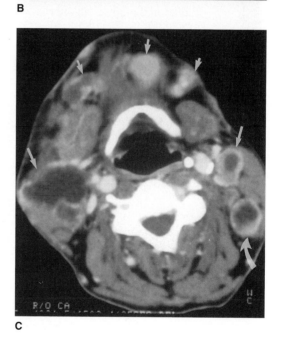

C

## Suggested Reading

Van der Brekel MW, Stel HV, Castelijns JA, et al. Cervical lymph node metastasis: assessment of radiologic criteria. *Radiology* 1990;177:379.

# *Nasopharyngeal Angiofibroma*

### KEY FACTS

- Nasopharyngeal angiofibroma is a histologically benign but locally aggressive tumor that occurs almost exclusively among boys (hence, "juvenile").

- All tumors originate near the pterygopalatine (90%) or sphenopalatine fossa, which may be expanded.

- Common clinical symptoms include nasal obstruction, epistaxis, facial deformities, anosmia, and headache.

- Extension in the maxillary and ethmoid sinuses is not uncommon (30% to 40%); intracranial extension is less common (5% to 10%).

- This tumor is almost exclusively fed by ipsilateral internal maxillary and ascending pharyngeal arteries.

- Differential diagnosis includes lymphoma, lymphoepithelioma, neurogenic tumor, soft-tissue sarcoma, hemangioma, polyp, and meningioma.

- Embolization followed by surgical intervention is the treatment of choice; radiation therapy is an alternative method.

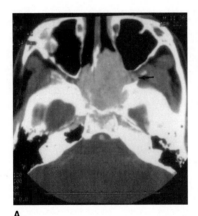 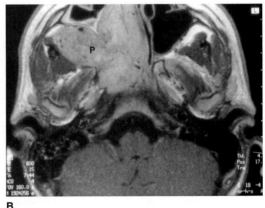

A                              B

FIGURE 27-12          (A) Axial postcontrast CT scan shows predominantly nasopharyngeal enhancing angiofibroma with mild extension into the left pterygopalatine fossa (*arrow*). (B) Axial postcontrast T1-weighted MR image of a different patient shows large enhancing angiofibroma in the right nasal cavity with a large component in an expanded pterygopalatine fossa (*P*).

### Suggested Reading

Garcia-Cervignon E, Bien S, Rufenacht D, et al. Pre-operative embolization of naso-pharyngeal angiofibromas: report of 58 cases. *Neuroradiology* 1988;30:556.

# *Glomus Jugulare*

## KEY FACTS

- Paragangliomas are derived from neural crest cells; most are histologically benign, but less than 6% show malignant growth.

- These tumors are more common among women 40 to 60 years of age.

- The most common locations include the carotid body, jugular bulb, and cochlear promontory, but the tumor may occur anywhere in the body.

- Glomus jugulare characteristically erodes the jugular foramen, enhances intensely, and contains calcifications and multiple flow voids (salt-and-pepper appearance if larger than 2.5 cm in diameter).

- The lesion usually presents with pulsatile tinnitus (remember that it may extend into the tympanic cavity) and jugular foramen syndrome (involvement of ninth, tenth, and eleventh cranial nerves).

- About 3% are multicentric, except in familial paragangliomas, when as many as 25% are multicentric.

- After radiation therapy these tumors show stabilization or reduction in size, decreased enhancement, and diminished flow voids.

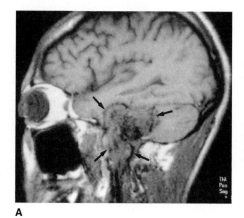 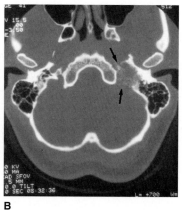

**A**   **B**

**FIGURE 27-13**   **(A)** Noncontrast parasagittal T1-weighted MR image shows glomus jugulare tumor (*arrows*) that contains multiple flow voids centrally. **(B)** Axial CT scan (bone window settings) of a different patient shows erosion (*arrows*) of the left jugular foramen by paraganglioma.

## Suggested Reading

Van Gils APG, van der Berg R, Falke THM, et al. MR diagnosis of paraganglioma of the head and neck: value of contrast enhancement. *Am J Roentgenol* 1994;162:147.

# *Hemangioma*

### KEY FACTS

- Hemangioma is a slow flow vascular malformation.
- It is the most common airway and parotid mass among children; it also may occur anywhere in the neck (e.g., muscles, temporal bone, or paranasal cavities) and orbits.
- Among young children, most of these lesions are capillary hemangiomas, and they may involute with age.
- Cavernous hemangiomas tend to occur after 16 years of age and do not involute with age.
- Hemangiomas present as soft masses that increase in size with Valsalva's maneuver (crying by children) or during pregnancy; an overlying skin hemangioma may be present.
- Hemangiomas involute by means of fatty infiltration.

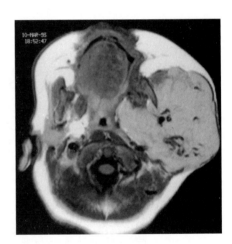

**FIGURE 27-14**
Axial postcontrast T1-weighted MR image shows large hemangioma predominantly in the masticator space. Note large vessels within the mass.

## Suggested Reading
Baker LL, Dillon WP, Hieshima GB, et al. Hemangiomas and vascular malformations of head and neck: MR characterization. *Am J Neuroradiol* 1993;14:307.

# *Lymphangioma*

## KEY FACTS

- Lymphangioma includes cystic hygroma, lymphangioma simplex, and cavernous lymphangioma.

- These benign, nonencapsulated masses contain large dilated spaces filled with milky fluid.

- About 75% of all lymphangiomas occur in the neck, and as many as 10% extend into the mediastinum.

- About 50% of lesions are present at birth, and most are found before 2 years of age; among adults about 30% of cystic neck masses are benign and related to lymphangioma.

- Most lesions occur in the posterior triangle of the neck, but they may be found in the floor of the mouth or submandibular region.

- Lymphangioma may be associated with systemic lymphatic abnormalities.

- At CT or MRI lymphangioma may be found to contain fluid levels caused by hemorrhage and the presence of unclotted blood.

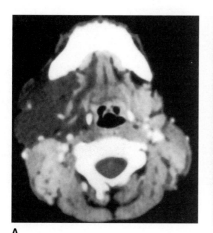 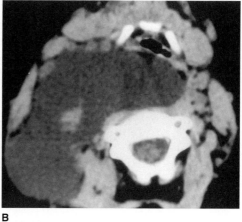

A                                    B

**FIGURE 27-15**    (A) Axial postcontrast CT scan shows cystic nonenhancing lymphangioma predominantly in the right submandibular space. (B) Inferiorly the lymphangioma involves the posterior triangle and retropharyngeal regions.

## Suggested Reading

Zadvinskis DP, Benson MT, Kerr HH, et al. Congenital malformations of the cervico-thoracic lymphatic system: embryology and pathogenesis. *Radiographics* 1992;12:1175.

# Branchial Cleft Cyst

## KEY FACTS

- Branchial cleft cysts represent incomplete proliferation, migration, or obliteration of one of the four branchial clefts.

- *First branchial cleft cysts* (8%) occur in the vicinity of the external auditory canal (may drain into it) or in the anterior triangle of the neck inferior to the mandible.

- *Second branchial cleft cysts* (>90%) occur in the anterior triangle at midneck, cross the common carotid artery bifurcation, and end at the palatine tonsil.

- *Third branchial cleft cysts* are uncommon, arise from the pyriform sinus, and are located anterior to the sternocleidomastoid muscle in the lower neck.

- *Fourth branchial cleft cysts* are very rare; they arise from the pyriform sinus, may extend caudal and behind the aortic arch or cephalad and posterior to the carotid artery; most are left-sided.

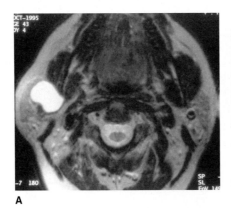 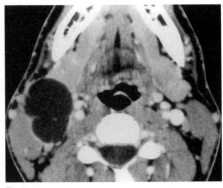

A                B

**FIGURE 27-16**  **(A)** Axial T2-weighted MR image shows cystic mass in right parotid gland. This mass extended superiorly to the external auditory canal making it a type 1 branchial cleft cyst. **(B)** Axial postcontrast CT scan of a different patient shows a type 2 branchial cleft anterior to the right sternocleidomastoid muscle.

### Suggested Reading
Benson MT, Dalen K, Mancuso AA, et al. Congenital anomalies of the branchial apparatus: embryology and pathologic anatomy. *Radiographics* 1992;12:943.

# *Thyroglossal Duct Cyst*

## KEY FACTS

- Thyroglossal duct cyst is the most common midline mass among children.
- Locations include below the hyoid bone (65%), suprahyoid (20%), and the level of the hyoid bone (15%).
- These cysts measure 2 to 4 cm in diameter and may enlarge progressively. Sudden enlargement may be associated with upper respiratory infection. Carcinoma occurs in 1% of cysts and is related to the presence of ectopic thyroid tissue.
- At imaging thyroglossal duct cysts are uni- or multilocular masses centered in the strap muscles with peripheral enhancement; the hyoid bone may contain a midline cleft.

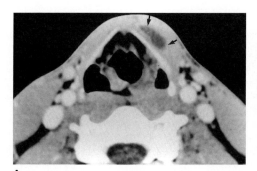 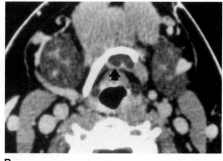

A                                                     B

**FIGURE 27-17**     **(A)** Axial postcontrast CT scan shows cyst mass (*arrows*) embedded in the left strap muscles. **(B)** At the level of the hyoid bone, the cyst (*arrow*) courses superiorly and is located posteriorly.

## Suggested Reading

Lanzieri CF. Head and neck case of the day: thyroglossal duct cyst. *Am J Roentgenol* 1997; 169:279.

## *Thyroid Masses*

### KEY FACTS

- Most thyroid masses are benign adenomas (but cannot be differentiated from small carcinomas), colloid cysts, or multinodular goiter.

- The most common carcinomas include papillary (>50%, which has the best prognosis), follicular (20%), medullary (10%), anaplastic (>5%, worst prognosis), and Hürthle cell (>2%).

- Lymphoma is not unusual; some patients have a history of thyroiditis.

- Both lymphoma and anaplastic carcinoma tend to invade the trachea.

- MRI with contrast medium is the ideal imaging method. If iodinated contrast medium for CT is given, it is preferable to wait 6 weeks before attempting a technetium-99m scan or 3 to 6 months before attempting a scan, uptake, or treatment with radioiodine.

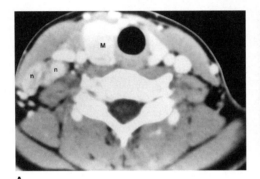 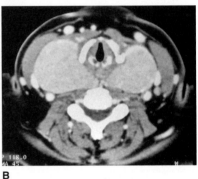

A                                           B

**FIGURE 27-18**    **(A)** Axial postcontrast CT scan shows dominant mass (*M*) in the right lobe of the thyroid. Note enlarged nodes (*n*) at level 5 on same side as mass. This proved to be mixed adenocarcinoma with metastases. **(B)** Axial postcontrast CT scan shows diffuse enlargement of the thyroid compatible with a multinodular goiter.

### Suggested Reading

Nakahara J, Noguchi S, Murakami N, et al. Gadolinium-enhanced MR imaging of thyroid and parathyroid masses. *Radiology* 1997;202:765.

# Sialolithiasis

### KEY FACTS

- The most common location for stones are Wharton's duct of the submandibular glands (80%), Stensen's duct of the parotid gland (10% to 15%), and the sublingual glands (>5%).

- Most stones are solitary and radiopaque.

- Stones cause acute sialoadenitis and abscess formation.

- Stones may be missed at MRI; therefore if an inflammatory process is considered, CT is best. If a tumor of the salivary gland is suspected, MRI is the ideal imaging method.

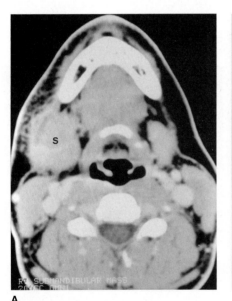

**A**

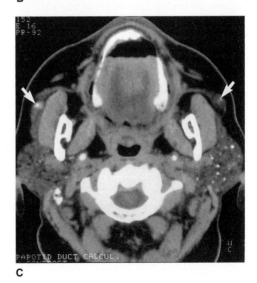

**B**

**C**

### FIGURE 27-19

(A) Axial postcontrast CT scan shows enlarged right submandibular gland (*S*) with reticulation of the adjacent fat and thickening of overlying skin. (B) Axial CT scan (bone window settings) of the same patient shows a large stone (*arrow*) in the right Wharton's duct. Smaller satellite calculi are present. (C) Axial CT scan of a different patient shows multiple small calculi in the parotid glands and in Stensen's ducts (*arrows*).

### Suggested Reading

Avrahami E, Englender M, Chen E, Shabtav D, Katz R, Harell M. CT of submandibular gland sialolithiasis. *Neuroradiology* 1996;38:287.

# Tornwaldt's Cyst

### KEY FACTS

- Tornwaldt's cysts represent a remnant of the notochordal bursa and are found among approximately 4% of the population.

- The cysts are located in the superoposterior nasopharynx centrally between the longus capiti muscles (occasionally they may be eccentric).

- The cysts almost always are incidental findings; but they may cause abscesses, halitosis, and a sore throat.

- The cysts usually measure 1 to 5 mm in diameter (in rare instances they may be as large as 3 cm in diameter) and contain highly proteinaceous fluid, which may produce high signal intensity on both T1-weighted and T2-weighted MR images.

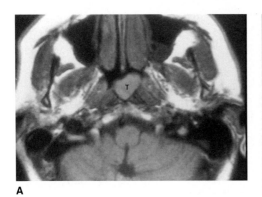

**A**

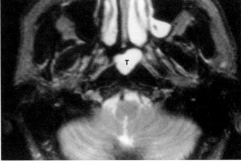

**B**

**FIGURE 27-20**

**(A)** Axial T1-weighted MR image shows slightly hyperintense (increased protein?) Tornwaldt's cyst (*T*) in nasopharynx. **(B)** On a corresponding T2-weighted image, the cyst (*T*) is bright. **(C)** Postcontrast axial CT scan of a different patient shows Tornwaldt's cyst (*arrows*) with minimal enhancement of its walls.

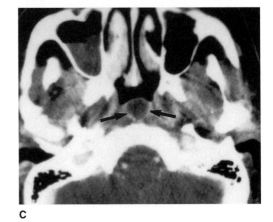

**C**

### Suggested Reading

Ford WJ, Brooks BS, el Gammal T. Thornwald cyst: an incidental MR diagnosis. *Am J Neuroradiol* 1987;8:922.

# 28 Paranasal Sinus Pathology

## Ostiomeatal Unit, Obstruction

### KEY FACTS

- The ostiomeatal unit (OMU) is formed by the following components:
- *Uncinate process:* thin bony lamina belonging to the ethmoid bone; it begins anteriorly at the lacrimal bone and extends posteriorly to the inferior nasal concha.
- *Ethmoidal infundibulum:* air space superolateral to the uncinate process and inferior to the ethmoidal bulla.
- *Semilunar hiatus:* air space above the uncinate process and inferior to the ethmoidal bulla communicating the infundibulum with the middle meatus.
- *Ostia* for the maxillary, anterior and middle ethmoidal complex, and frontal recess form the medial aspect of infundibulum.
- The OMU is commonly obstructed by mucosal thickening, polyps, an enlarged or pneumatized uncinate process, deviated nasal septum with or without spurs, concha bullosa of the middle turbinate, large ethmoid bullae, and paradoxic middle turbinates.

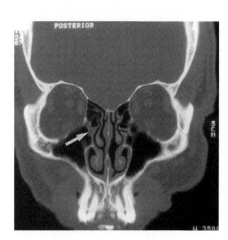

**FIGURE 28-1**
Coronal CT scan shows small polypoid soft tissue (*arrow*) obstructing the infundibulum of the right ostiomeatal unit.

### Suggested Reading

Mafee MF, Chow JM, Meyers R. Functional endoscopic sinus surgery: anatomy, CT screening, indications, and complications. *Am J Roentgenol* 1993;160:735.

# Developmental Anomalies of the Ostiomeatal Unit

## KEY FACTS

- Developmental anomalies of the nasal cavity include concha bullosa, paradoxic middle turbinates, septal deviation, enlarged ethmoid bullae, and Haller cells.

- Concha bullosa (extramural middle turbinal cells) is present among 30% to 50% of the population; if large, the lesion may deviate the nasal septum or become superinfected (concha bullitis); if the ostium is occluded, a mucocele may form.

- Paradoxic middle turbinates are common. They are diagnosed when their curvature is the reverse of the curvature of the inferior turbinates; if small, paradoxic middle turbinates are usually bilateral; if large, they are unilateral and may produce septal deviation.

- Hypoplasia of the middle turbinates is uncommon and does not produce symptoms.

- Enlarged ethmoid bullae or Haller cells may result in obstruction of the ipsi- or contralateral infundibula.

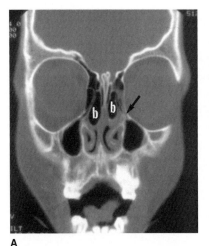 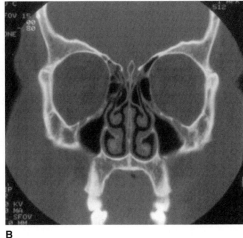

A                                              B

**FIGURE 28-2**

**(A)** Coronal CT scan shows bilateral concha bullosa (*b*) involving the middle turbinates. The left-sided lesion narrows the infundibulum (*arrow*). **(B)** Coronal CT scan of a different patient shows paradoxic course of both middle turbinates. This anomaly does not result in compromise of the ostiomeatal units.

## Suggested Reading

Earwaker J. Anatomic variants in sinonasal CT. *Radiographics* 1993;13:381.

# *Mucous Retention Cysts*

KEY FACTS

- Mucous retention cysts generally are the sequelae of inflammatory sinusitis, allergy, or trauma.
- The cysts represent obstruction of a minor salivary gland or a mucus-secreting gland.
- They occur among more than 10% of the population, most commonly in the maxillary sinus.
- These cysts usually are incidental and asymptomatic findings.
- If small, the cysts have an upward convex border; if large, the superior surface becomes flattened, and the cyst may simulate a fluid level; if very large, a cyst may obstruct the sinus ostia.
- Caution: among adults, early paranasal sinus carcinoma may appear identical to a mucous retention cyst.
- As with most inflammatory sinus disease, retention cysts are bright on T2-weighted magnetic resonance (MR) images.

*(continued)*

# *Mucous Retention Cysts* (Continued)

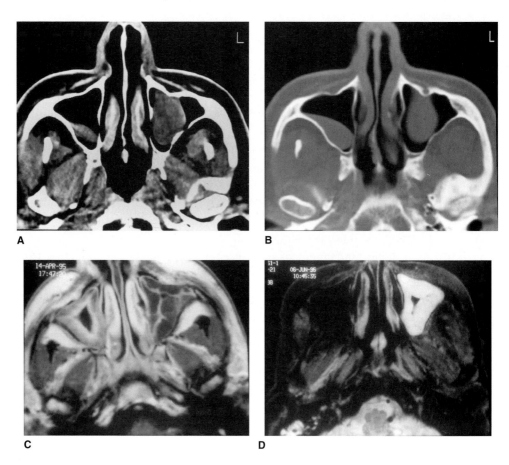

A

B

C

D

**FIGURE 28-3**    **(A)** Axial CT scan shows low density in mucous retention cysts in the maxillary sinuses. **(B)** CT scan of the same patient with corresponding bone window settings shows the cysts and mild thickening of the lateral wall of the right maxillary sinus. **(C)** Axial postcontrast T1-weighted MR image of a different patient shows thick, enhancing mucosa in right maxillary sinus and multiple submucosal retention cysts of low signal intensity in the left maxillary sinus. **(D)** Two months after conservative therapy, an axial T2-weighted MR image of the same patient as in C shows resolution of thick mucosa in right maxillary sinus but persistent hyperintense cysts in the left antrum.

## Suggested Reading

Som PM, Shapiro MD, Biller HF, Sasaki C, Lawson W. Sinonasal tumor and inflammatory tissues: differentiation with MR imaging. *Radiology* 1988;167:803.

# *Sinonasal Polyps*

KEY FACTS

- Polyps are usually the sequelae of inflammation, vasomotor or infectious rhinitis, diabetes, and cystic fibrosis.
- Polyps are uncommon among children in the absence of cystic fibrosis. They are found among 4% of the population, are more common in men, and asthma is an important predisposing factor.
- Polyps may occur in any sinus (but are more common in the maxillary sinus). They may enlarge and become a conglomerate mass, which expands the sinuses and the infundibula, may erode their septa, or may result in loss of bone density in the ethmoid trabeculae, turbinates, and nasal septum.
- Polyps occasionally behave aggressively and erode bone (producing intracranial extension).
- Polyps may protrude from a sinus into the nasal cavities (antrochonal and sphenochoanal polyps).
- Polyps may be infected with fungi (generally *Aspergillus* organisms). Computed tomographic (CT) scans may show high density or calcifications (25% to 50%) caused by calcium phosphate and calcium sulfate in necrotic mycetoma.
- Infarcted polyps may be hyperdense on noncontrast CT scans. The presence of low T2 signal intensity does not imply malignant growth but correlates with the presence of desiccated secretions or fungal infection.

*(continued)*

## *Sinonasal Polyps* *(Continued)*

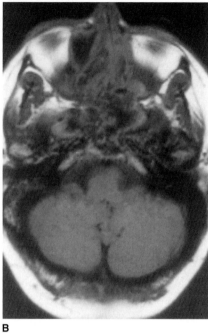

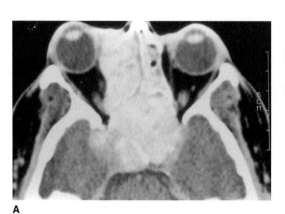

A                                                B

**FIGURE 28-4**    **(A)** Axial postcontrast CT scan shows high-density expansile and extensive sinonasal polyposis. There is extension into the right orbit, sella, and cavernous sinuses. **(B)** Noncontrast T1-weighted MR image of the same patient shows the polyps to be mostly of low signal intensity, which could be confused with normal aeration.

### Suggested Reading

Zinreich SJ, Kennedy DW, Malar J, et al. Fungal sinusitis: diagnosis with CT and MR imaging. *Radiology* 1988;169:439.

# Acute (Uncomplicated) Sinusitis

## KEY FACTS

- The most common causes of acute uncomplicated sinusitis are viral upper respiratory tract infection—bacterial, allergic, and fungal.
- Although fluid levels are the most common manifestation, they actually occur in less than 50% of cases. Fluid levels also occur with trauma (hemorrhage), intubation, barotrauma, and bleeding disorders.
- A fluid level in the frontal sinus is most specific for infectious sinusitis.
- A fluid level in the sphenoid sinus may be associated with a fracture of the base of the skull with cerebrospinal fluid (CSF) leakage.
- Among older adults, a solitary opacified (or with fluid level) paranasal sinus should raise the possibility of an underlying tumor.
- Fluid levels in the presence of nasal or oral tubes are not diagnostic for infection.

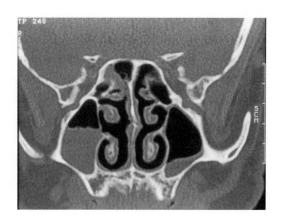

**FIGURE 28-5**
Coronal CT scan shows fluid level in the right maxillary sinus and polypoid mucosa in the alveolar recess of the left maxillary sinus.

## Suggested Reading

Yousem DM. Imaging of sinonasal inflammatory disease. *Radiology* 1993;188:303.

# *Fungal Sinusitis*

KEY FACTS

- Aspergillosis (among healthy patients) and mucormycosis (among immunodepressed patients) are the most common causes of fungal sinusitis (others include candidiasis, histoplasmosis, cryptococcus infection, and coccidioidomycosis).
- The maxillary and ethmoid sinuses are most commonly involved; isolated involvement of the sphenoid sinus suggests aspergillosis.
- This type of sinusitis may occur in the setting of sinonasal polyposis.
- Aspergillosis may cause a vasculitis, mycotic aneurysms, and vessel thrombosis.
- Mucormycosis may involve the orbits and cavernous sinuses.
- Secretions of high density on plain films or CT scans (calcification is seen on CT scans in 50% of cases) and of low signal intensity on MR images suggest the diagnosis.

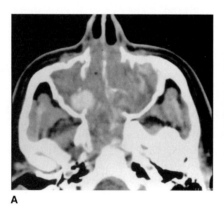 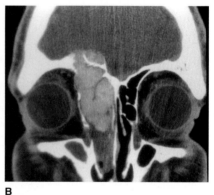

A                                                 B

FIGURE  28-6      (A) Axial CT scan shows extensive sinonasal polyposis with bone destruction. Areas of high density within the lesion suggest superimposed fungal infection. (B) Coronal CT scan of a different patient shows high-density polyposis (caused by aspergillosis) expanding the right ethmoid complex and destroying the roof of the orbit because of extension into the supraorbital recess of the ethmoid sinus.

## Suggested Reading

Ashdown BC, Tien RD, Felsberg GJ. Aspergillosis of the brain and paranasal sinuses in immuno-compromised patients: CT and MR imaging findings. *Am J Roentgenol* 1994;162:155.

# *Malignant Tumors of the Paranasal Sinuses*

## KEY FACTS

- Squamous cell carcinoma is the most common malignant tumor (80%); advanced local disease is common at diagnosis; the maxillary sinus is most commonly affected; 20% of patients have nodal metastases at diagnosis.

- Undifferentiated carcinoma and lymphoma are uncommon and are indistinguishable at imaging from squamous cell carcinoma.

- Adenoid cystic carcinoma accounts for 10% of sinonasal malignant tumors, involves the ethmoid sinuses more often, and initially may have a benign appearance.

- Primary sarcoma (e.g., osteosarcoma and chondrosarcoma) is a rare and destructive tumor that contains calcifications on CT scans.

- Many malignant tumors of the paranasal sinuses have low signal intensity on T2-weighted MR images; differential diagnosis for this appearance includes air, desiccated secretions, fungal infections (calcium), hemorrhage, bone, and enamel.

- Processes that simulate carcinoma include mucormycosis, Wegener's granulomatosis (and midline granuloma), and cocaine abuse.

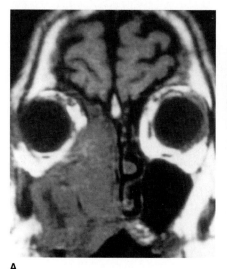

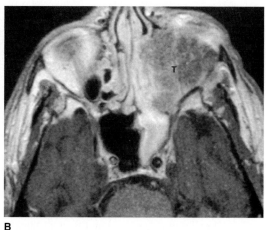

**A**   **B**

**FIGURE 28-7**   (A) Coronal noncontrast T1-weighted MR image shows mass of intermediate signal intensity in the right maxillary sinus eroding its floor and lateral walls. There is extension into the ipsilateral ethmoid complex and into the orbit. (B) Axial T2-weighted MR image of the same patient shows the tumor (*T*) to be relatively hypointense. Note bright inflammatory secretions in the right-sided compartment of the sphenoid sinus.

## Suggested Reading

Allbery SM, Chaljub G, Cho NL, Rassekh CH, John SD, Guinto FC. MR imaging of nasal masses. *Radiographics* 1995;15:1311.

# *Mucocele*

## KEY FACTS

- The most common cause of expanded sinuses with thinned walls, mucoceles are produced by obstruction of ostia or of individual sinus compartments from chronic inflammation or allergies (as well as trauma and underlying tumors).

- Locations include the frontal (65%), ethmoid (25%), maxillary (10%), and sphenoid sinuses (2%).

- Facial deformity is the most common initial symptom; the presence of pain should suggest the possibility of superimposed infection (mucopyocele).

- Most mucoceles are of low signal intensity on T1-weighted MR images and hyperintense on T2-weighted images; inspissated mucoceles are hypointense on both T1-weighted and T2-weighted MR images and may simulate dilated but aerated sinuses.

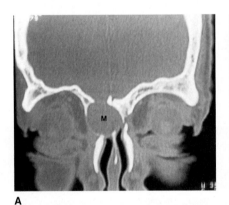 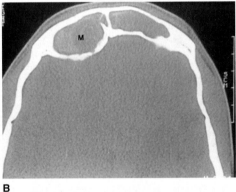

**A**                    **B**

FIGURE 28-8    **(A)** Coronal CT scan shows mucocele (*M*) with expansion of the right frontoethmoidal region. **(B)** Axial CT scan of a different patient shows mucocele (*M*) resulting in expansion of the right-sided compartment of the frontal sinus. The left-sided compartment of this sinus is opacified but not expanded.

## Suggested Reading

Van Tassel P, Lee YY, Jing BS, et al. Mucoceles of the paranasal sinuses: MR imaging with CT correlation. *Am J Neuroradiol* 1989;10:607.

# *Papilloma*

## KEY FACTS

- Papilloma is rare. It constitutes 4% of all sinonasal tumors. The tumor arises from a special type of epithelium (ciliated columnar with mucous Bowman's glands) at sinonasal cavities (schneiderian papilloma).

- More than 50% of papillomas arise from the nasal septum and are called *fungiform papilloma*.

- About 47% are inverting papillomas that arise in the lateral nasal wall and extend (invert) into the adjacent maxillary and ethmoid sinuses or, less commonly, into the sphenoid, cribiform plate, and frontal sinuses.

- About 3% are cylindric cell papillomas (similar in location to inverting ones).

- Papilloma tends to be unilateral.

- Associated malignant tumor (mainly squamous cell carcinoma) is found in 3% to 24% of papillomas and tends to be seen more commonly with the inverting type (although this is controversial).

- En bloc removal of the lesion is the goal because imaging cannot help one differentiate benign from malignant lesions.

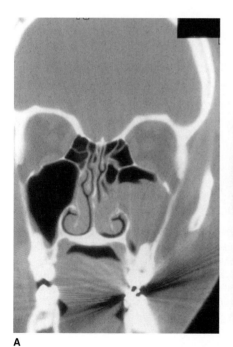
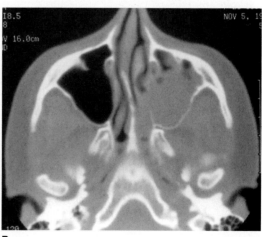

A    B

**FIGURE 28-9** (A) Coronal CT scan shows papilloma almost completely filling the left maxillary sinus. The lesion has extended into the ipsilateral nasal cavity through widening of an accessory ostium. (B) Axial CT scan of the same patient shows mass in left maxillary sinus extending through the medial wall into the ipsilateral nasal cavity.

## Suggested Reading

Roobottom CA, Jewell FM, Kabala J. Primary and recurrent inverting papilloma: appearances with magnetic resonance imaging. *Clin Radiol* 1995;50:472.

# Fibroosseous Lesions of Sinonasal Cavities

### KEY FACTS

- Osteomas are zones of compact bone in the frontal and ethmoid sinuses or any facial bone; they may be caused by infection or trauma. Most are asymptomatic, but some lesions cause headaches and occasionally produce obstructive sinusitis. These lesions are more common among persons 15 to 40 years of age.
- Osteoid osteoma occasionally arises in the frontal or ethmoid region.
- Osteoblastoma may occur in the maxilla, frontal, or sphenoethmoidal region.
- Monostotic fibrous dysplasia (more common) involves the maxilla or mandible in 20% to 25% of instances; polyostotic fibrous dysplasia (less common) occurs almost exclusively among women and involves the skull and facial bones in 40% to 60% of instances.
- Fibrous dysplasia encroaches sinonasal cavities and neurovascular foramina.
- Malignant degeneration occurs among less than 1% of patients with fibrous dysplasia (osteosarcoma, fibrosarcoma, and chondrosarcoma).

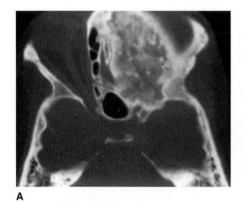 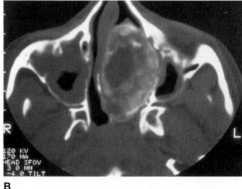

A                                                            B

FIGURE 28-10    (A) Axial CT scan shows fibrous dysplasia involving the roof of the left orbit, ethmoid sinuses, greater sphenoidal wing, and sphenoid sinus. (B) Axial CT scan of a different patient shows large ossifying fibroma expanding the left nasal cavity. There is thickened mucosa in both maxillary sinuses (right > left).

### Suggested Reading

Jee WH, Choi KH, Choe BY, Park JM, Shinn KS. Fibrous dysplasia: MR imaging characteristics with radiopathologic correlation. *Am J Roentgenol* 1996;167:1523.

# 29  Temporal Bone and Temporomandibular Joint

## *Temporal Bone Fracture, Longitudinal*

### KEY FACTS

- Longitudinal fractures are the most common (70% to 80%) temporal bone fractures; they result from blows to the temporoparietal region.
- These fractures may produce conductive hearing loss caused by ossicular chain dislocation (the most common are incudostapedial and malleoincudal dislocations).
- Consider incudostapedial dislocation when the distance between these ossicles is more than 2 mm.
- Consider malleoincudal dislocation if any distance exists between these two ossicles.
- The tympanic membrane often is perforated.
- Facial palsy (10% to 20%) is delayed (because of swelling of the descending facial nerve and entrapment within the bone canal) and generally resolves spontaneously.
- There is an increased incidence of postfracture cholesteatoma.
- Air in the temporomandibular joint is an indirect sign of temporal bone fracture.
- Disruption of the tegmen tympani with subsequent leakage of cerebrospinal fluid (CSF) is a well-known complication.

*(continued)*

# *Temporal Bone Fracture, Longitudinal* *(Continued)*

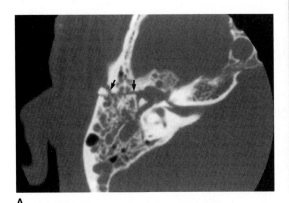

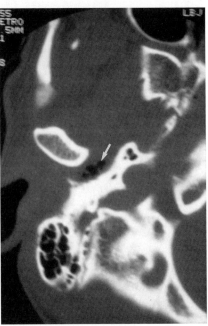

A                                                        B

**FIGURE 29-1**   **(A)** Axial CT scan shows longitudinal fracture (*arrows*) of right temporal bone. The head of the malleolus is not depicted, a finding compatible with malleoincudal dislocation. The middle ear is opacified. **(B)** Axial CT scan of a different patient with temporal bone fracture shows air (*arrow*) in the right temporomandibular joint.

## Suggested Reading

Betz BW, Wiener MD. Air in the temporomandibular joint fossa: CT sign of temporal bone fracture. *Radiology* 1991;180:463.

# *Temporal Bone Fracture, Transverse*

## KEY FACTS

- Transverse fractures are the second most common (10% to 20%) type of temporal bone fracture (but some authors believe that mixed or complex fractures are more common than either longitudinal or transverse fractures).

- These fractures result from frontal or occipital blows.

- They produce sensorineural hearing loss and vertigo caused by involvement of the otic capsule or transection of the eighth cranial nerve (hearing deficits produced in the absence of fracture crossing the otic capsule are probably caused by labyrinthine concussion).

- Facial palsy is more common with transverse fractures than with longitudinal fractures and usually is permanent because it is caused by transection of the nerve.

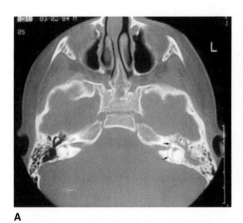 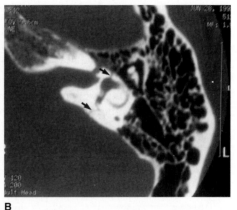

A          B

**FIGURE 29-2**    **(A)** Axial CT scan shows a transverse fracture (*arrows*) crossing the basal turn of the cochlea and fundus of the left internal auditory canal. **(B)** Axial CT scan of a different patient shows transverse fracture (*arrows*) crossing the left vestibule.

## Suggested Reading

Holland BA, Brant-Zawadski M. High resolution CT of temporal bone trauma. *Am J Neuroradiol* 1984;5:291.

# *Vestibular Schwannoma*

## KEY FACTS

- Vestibular schwannoma is the most common posterior fossa tumor among adults and is the second most common intracranial extraaxial tumor after meningioma among adults.

- 75% to 80% of masses in the cerebellopontine angle cistern are vestibular schwannomas.

- The tumor arises from Scarpa's ganglion (glial-Schwann cell junction) in the superior division of the vestibular nerve.

- This tumor is more common among women between 40 and 60 years of age.

- Bilateral eighth nerve schwannomas are pathognomonic for neurofibromatosis type 2.

- The most common symptoms include sensorineural hearing loss, tinnitus, headache, and disequilibrium.

- Facial nerve palsy is uncommon because the seventh nerve is fairly resistant to pressure.

- About 5% to 22% of vestibular schwannomas are atypical at imaging and have associated arachnoid cysts or central necrosis or are partially or completely cystic.

- Differential diagnosis includes mainly meningioma, metastasis, sarcoidosis, paraganglioma, and chordoma.

- Initial screening may be performed with only constructive interference in the steady state (CISS) images; after surgical intervention contrast-enhanced magnetic resonance imaging (MRI) is needed.

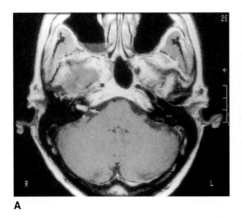
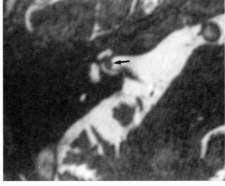

A                                                   B

**FIGURE 29-3**　　(A) Postcontrast T1-weighted MR image shows enhancing intracanalicular vestibular schwannoma (*arrow*). (B) Axial CISS MR image of a different patient shows tiny vestibular schwannoma (*arrow*) in the fundus of the right internal auditory canal.

## Suggested Reading

Lhuillier FM, Doyon DL, Halimi PM, Sigal RC, Sterkers JM. Magnetic resonance imaging of acoustic neuromas: pitfalls and differential diagnosis. *Neuroradiology* 1992;34:144.

# Facial Nerve Schwannoma

### KEY FACTS

- Facial nerve schwannoma accounts for only 5% of all facial nerve palsies (the remainder are of viral or posttraumatic causation).

- The onset of facial nerve palsy is slow and progressive.

- These tumors tend to arise in the geniculate ganglion but may involve any of its segments.

- Identification of extension along the labyrinthine segment of the facial nerve is important in making the correct presurgical diagnosis.

- Differential diagnosis includes facial nerve hemangioma, vestibular schwannoma, viral neuritis (Bell's palsy and Ramsay Hunt syndrome), and meningioma.

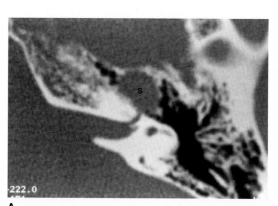
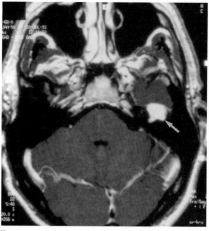

**FIGURE 29-4** **(A)** Axial CT scan shows mass (*s*) involving the left geniculate ganglion. **(B)** Postcontrast axial T1-weighted MR image of the same patient shows the tumor (*arrow*) to enhance homogeneously.

### Suggested Reading

Swartz JD, Harnsberger HR. *Imaging of the temporal bone.* 3rd ed. New York: Thieme Medical Publishers, 1998:370.

# *Bell's Palsy*

### KEY FACTS

- Bell's palsy is characterized by acute onset and spontaneous resolution within 4 to 6 months.

- Possible causes include viral infection, ischemia, immunologic disorders, and polyneuropathy associated with other central nervous system (CNS) or systemic disorders.

- About 15% of patients have an atypical course characterized by slow progression and no remission.

- Only 1% to 5% of all facial nerve palsies are bilateral and are most often viral in nature.

- MRI shows enhancement of the seventh nerve, but the degree of enhancement has no correlation with the severity of clinical findings and does not help one predict outcome.

- Enhancement of the descending portion of the facial nerve is a normal finding seen in 76% of magnetic resonance (MR) studies because of the presence of a rich circumneural vascular plexus.

- Differential diagnosis includes Ramsay Hunt syndrome (caused by herpes zoster infection), sarcoidosis, Lyme disease, lymphoma, perineural tumor spread, and early facial nerve schwannoma.

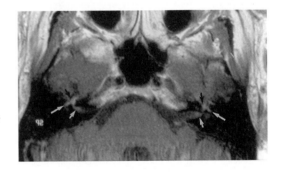

**FIGURE 29-5**

Axial postcontrast T1-weighted MR image shows enhancement of both facial nerves in the fundi of the internal auditory canals (*short white arrows*), geniculate ganglia (*black arrows*), and proximal horizontal portions (*long white arrows*).

## Suggested Reading

Sartoretti-Schefer S, Wichman W, Valvanis A. Idiopathic, herpetic, and HIV-associated facial nerve palsies: abnormal MR enhancement patterns. *Am J Neuroradiol* 1994;5:479.

# Vestibular Aqueduct Syndrome

## KEY FACTS

- Less than 1% of patients with congenital sensorineural hearing loss have abnormalities detected with imaging studies.

- The vestibular aqueduct syndrome is the most commonly recognized cause of congenital hearing loss.

- The normal vestibular aqueduct extends from the vestibule to the posterior aspect of the petrous bone and contains the endolymphatic duct the function of which is equilibration of endolymphatic fluid pressure.

- In the vestibular aqueduct syndrome, computed tomography (CT) shows dilatation of the vestibular aqueduct (as a rule the vestibular aqueduct should be no wider than a semicircular canal or more than 1.5 mm at its midpoint).

- A large vestibular aqueduct may be associated with cochlear anomalies (from Mondini dysplasia to absence of the modiolus).

- Enlargement of the endolymphatic sac may occur in the presence of a normal-sized aqueduct and it may present as a mass in the cerebellopontine angle region.

- Other causes of congenital hearing loss are trauma, metabolic disorders, viral infection, Michel's syndrome, Mondini dysplasia, Scheibe's deafness, and Alexander's disease.

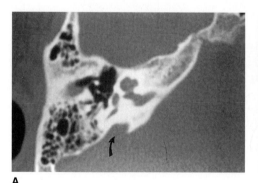
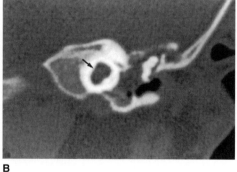

**A**   **B**

**FIGURE 29-6**   **(A)** Axial CT scan shows dilatation of the right vestibular aqueduct (*arrow*) and absence of the modiolus of the cochlea. **(B)** Coronal CT scan of a different patient with vestibular aqueduct syndrome shows that the left cochlea (*arrow*) is a single cavity without partitions or turns (Mondini dysplasia). The middle ear is opacified.

## Suggested Reading

Castillo M, Mukherji SK. Congenital malformations of the inner ear. In: *Imaging of the pediatric head, neck, and spine.* Philadelphia: Lippincott-Raven, 1996:443.

# Labyrinthitis Obliterans (Ossificans)

## KEY FACTS

- Labyrinthitis obliterans is an inflammatory process (possibly viral) that results in sensorineural hearing loss and vertigo in the acute period.
- Causes include tympanogenic, meningogenic (bacterial meningitis), hematogenic (viral), autoimmune, toxic, and posttraumatic (including iatrogenic) factors.
- Unilateral disease is usually tympanogenic in origin; bilateral disease is usually meningogenic or hematogenic in nature.
- CT scans show focal (round window or basilar turn of cochlea) or diffuse ossification of the membranous labyrinth (the cochlear and lateral semicircular canal promontories are preserved, but with congenital inner ear dysplasia this structure may not form).
- At MRI (particularly CISS images), the normal T2 brightness of the labyrinth is not well seen.

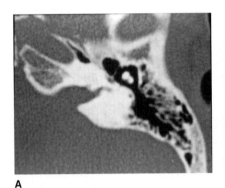 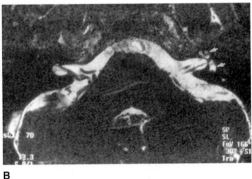

A        B

**FIGURE 29-7**     **(A)** Axial CT scan shows ossification of all structures belonging to the otic capsule (nonvisualization of the cochlea, vestibule, and semicircular canals). **(B)** Axial CISS MR image of a different patient shows normal endolymph in left cochlea and vestibule (*arrows*) and absence of this fluid in the right cochlea compatible with labyrinthitis obliterans. This finding prevents cochlear implantation on the affected side.

## Suggested Reading

Guirado CR, Martinez P, Roiq R, et al. Three-dimensional MR of the inner ear with steady-state free precession. *Am J Neuroradiol* 1995;16:1909.

# *Glomus Tympanicum*

### KEY FACTS

- Glomus tympanicum is a paraganglioma at the cochlear promontory that arises from the plexus formed by the nerves of Jacobson (tympanic branch of ninth cranial nerve) and Arnold (auricular ramus of tenth cranial nerve).

- This tumor generally occurs among women older than 30 years and is the most common tumor of the middle ear among adults.

- The most common symptoms include pulsatile tinnitus, hearing loss, and facial nerve palsy (30%).

- The blood supply is mostly through external carotid artery branches (especially the ascending pharyngeal artery); therefore presurgical embolization is relatively easy.

- Glomus tympanicum presents as a retrotympanic red mass. Differential diagnosis includes aberrant internal carotid artery, persistent stapedial artery, dehiscent jugular bulb (or diverticulum), cholesterol granuloma, or hemangioma.

- Only 2% of these tumors are multicentric (less than paragangliomas arising elsewhere).

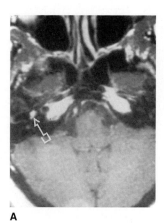 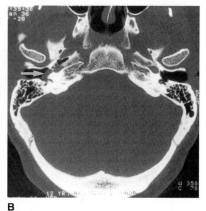

A              B

**FIGURE 29-8**     (A) Axial postcontrast T1-weighted MR image shows small and enhancing right glomus tympanicum tumor (*arrow*). (B) Axial CT scan of the same patient shows a small mass (*arrow*) overlying the cochlear promontory.

### Suggested Reading

Weissman JL, Hirsch BE. Beyond the promontory: the multifocal origin of glomus tympanicum tumors. *Am J Neuroradiol* 1998;19:119.

# *Vascular Anomalies, Middle Ear*

## KEY FACTS

- Vascular anomalies of the middle ear generally present as vascular retrotympanic masses that are indistinguishable from glomus tympanicum.

- Only seldom are these anomalies associated with conductive hearing loss.

- Jugular bulb variants include asymmetric jugular foramen (most common and generally on the right), high-riding jugular bulb (occurs among 6% of the population), dehiscent jugular bulb, and jugular bulb diverticulum.

- *Aberrant carotid artery* is a misnomer. It results from enlargement of the inferior tympanic artery as it anastomoses with a large caroticotympanic artery caused by regression of the cervical internal carotid artery (ICA). The presence of this anomaly may be confirmed with magnetic resonance angiography (MRA).

- Persistent stapedial artery is very rare and may be associated with an aberrant ICA. Characteristic imaging findings for persistent stapedial artery include absence of the foramen spinosum and enlarged tympanic portion of the facial nerve because this artery usually follows the course of the nerve.

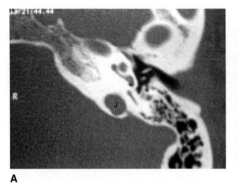

A

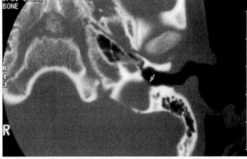

B

## FIGURE 29-9

(A) Axial CT scan shows incidentally found jugular bulb diverticulum (*J*) extending to the level of the basal turn of the cochlea. (B) Axial CT scan of a different patient shows absence of bone (dehiscence, *arrow*) between the left jugular bulb and the middle ear. (C) Coronal CT scan shows aberrant course of the left internal carotid artery (*arrow*) through the hypotympanic portion of the middle ear cavity.

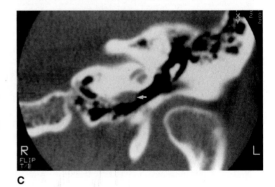

C

## Suggested Reading

Swartz JD, Harnsberger HR. *Imaging of the temporal bone*. 3rd ed. New York: Thieme Medical Publishers, 1998:187.

# *Cholesteatoma, Acquired (Secondary)*

## KEY FACTS

- Acquired cholesteatoma represents ingrowth of squamous epithelium through the tympanic membrane with deposition of cells and keratin debris in the middle ear.

- A mass-like lesion forms in the middle ear and erodes ossicles and bone.

- Pars flaccida cholesteatoma (most common type) begins in Prussak's space (therefore erodes the scutum) and extends to the epitympanum, aditus ad antrum, and mastoid antrum.

- Pars tensa cholesteatoma begins in the mesotympanum, involves the sinus tympani, and erodes the ossicles (which is the most common associated abnormality on CT scans).

- Complications include dehiscence of the tegmen tympani with intracranial extension (produces meningitis, venous thrombosis, abscess, or CSF leak), erosion of the labyrinth with development of a perilymphatic fistula, facial nerve palsy, hearing loss, and automastoidectomy (especially with mural cholesteatoma).

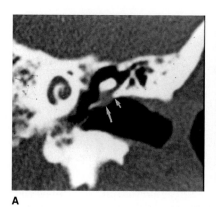
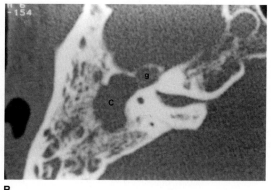

**A**     **B**

**FIGURE 29-10**     **(A)** Coronal CT scan shows cholesteatoma (*long arrow*) in Prussak's space. There is blunting of the tip (*short arrow*) of the scutum. **(B)** Axial CT scan of a different patient shows extensive cholesteatoma (*C*) eroding and expanding the right middle ear cavity. Note that the process has extended to involve the region of the geniculate ganglion (*g*).

## Suggested Reading

Ishii K, Takahashi S, Kobayashi T, Matsumoto K, Ishibashi T. MR imaging of middle ear cholesteatomas. *J Comput Assist Tomogr* 1991;15:934.

# *Cholesterol Granuloma*

### KEY FACTS

- Cholesterol granuloma also is known as *cyst of the petrous apex.*
- It results from obstruction (caused by Eustachian tube dysfunction) of an aerated petrous bone apex with accumulation of secretions and repeated hemorrhaging.
- This tumor occurs in association with chronic middle ear inflammation and is the most common lesion of the petrous apex.
- It presents with headache and fifth or sixth cranial nerve dysfunction, but many tumors are incidental findings.
- The granuloma is characteristically expansile and bright on both T1-weighted and T2-weighted MR images (resulting from the presence of cholesterol crystals).
- This tumor should not be confused with congenital cholesteatoma (epidermoid) of the petrous apex, which is usually of CSF-like signal intensity on MR images (however, epidermoids occasionally are bright and indistinguishable from the more common cholesterol granuloma).

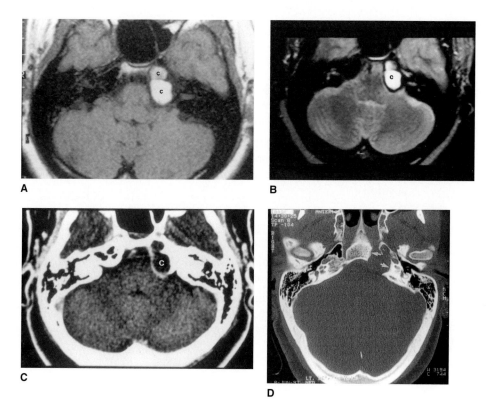

**FIGURE 29-11**

**(A)** Noncontrast axial T1-weighted MR image shows bright cholesterol cyst (*c*) in the apex of the left temporal pyramid. **(B)** Corresponding T2-weighted image shows the lesion (*c*) to be bright and surrounded by a rim of low signal intensity. **(C)** Axial CT scan of the same patient as in **B** shows the lesion (*c*) to be hypodense. **(D)** Axial CT scan (bone window settings) of a different patient shows smooth erosion (*arrows*) of the left petrous bone apex by a cholesterol cyst.

## Suggested Reading

Mafee MF, Kumar A, Heffner DK. Epidermoid cyst (cholesteatoma) and cholesterol granuloma of the temporal bone and epidermoid cysts affecting the brain. *Neuroimaging Clin North Am* 1994;4:561.

# Temporomandibular Joint, Dislocated Disc

### KEY FACTS

- Displacement of the disc is the most common cause of internal derangement of the temporomandibular joint (TMJ) and is more common among women during the third and fourth decades of life.

- Disc displacement *with* reduction is clinically characterized by normal opening of the mouth (although some limitation may be present) with a click in the last phase of closing the mouth as the disc reduces to normal position.

- Disc displacement *without* reduction is clinically characterized by limitation during mouth opening with slight mandibular deviation toward the affected side, and no click is present.

- If the disc is not seen on oblique sagittal MR images, obtain coronal images to exclude medial or lateral disc displacement.

- Late changes associated with disc displacement include disc deformities (including perforations, which are not seen on MR images), flattening of the condylar head, and fragmentation of the joint with multiple joint bone mice.

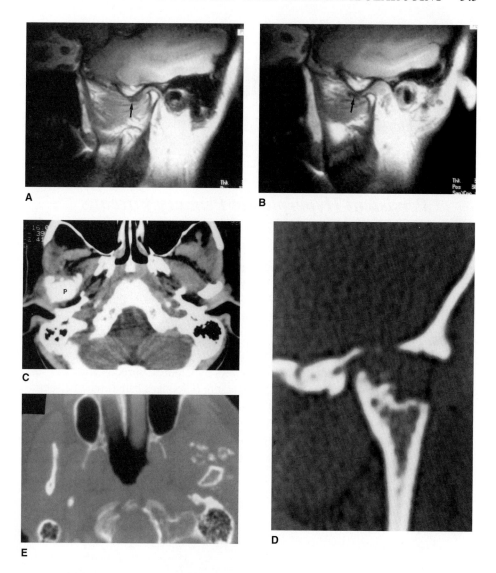

A

B

C

D

E

FIGURE 29-12     **(A)** Oblique parasagittal T1-weighted MR image shows disc (*arrow*) with anterior dislocation in the closed-mouth position. The condyle has a small osteophyte anteriorly. **(B)** Corresponding open-mouth view of the same patient shows incomplete anterior translation of the condyle and persistent (nonreduction) anterior dislocation of the disc (*arrow*). **(C)** Axial CT scan of a different patient shows hyperdense Proplast implant (*P*) in the right temporomandibular joint. **(D)** Coronal CT scan (bone window settings) of the same patient as in **C** shows erosion of the superior border of the joint by an inflammatory reaction elicited by the implant. **(E)** Axial CT scan of a different patient shows multiple bone fragments in the left temporomandibular joint, which in this instance were caused by pigmented villonodular synovitis.

## Suggested Reading

Tasaki MM, Westesson PL. Temporomandibular joint: diagnostic accuracy with sagittal and coronal MR imaging. *Radiology* 1993;186:723.

# 30   Orbital Pathology

## *Persistent Hyperplastic Primary Vitreous*

### KEY FACTS

- Persistent hyperplastic primary vitreous (PHPV) is a persistent, hyperplastic, embryonic hyaloid vascular system; patients may also have seizures, hearing loss, mental deficiencies, and cataracts.
- PHPV is the second most common cause of leukokoria after retinoblastoma.
- The affected eye is usually small (microphthalmia).
- Computed tomography (CT) shows hyperdense vitreous with no calcifications; a thin central structure (Cloquet's canal) may be seen extending from the posterior retina to the lens; the vitreous may enhance, and retinal detachments may be present.
- At magnetic resonance imaging (MRI), PHPV tends to be hyperintense on T2-weighted images, whereas retinoblastoma usually is hypointense.

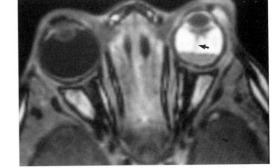

**FIGURE 30-1**
Axial T1-weighted MR image shows a small left eye containing a fluid level and a midline linear structure (*arrow*) representing Cloquet's canal. The fetal hyaloid artery courses in this structure. The lens is dysplastic.

### Suggested Reading
Kaste SC, Jenkins JJ, Myer D, Fontanesi J, Pratt CB. Persistent hyperplastic primary vitreous of the eye: imaging findings with pathologic correlation. *Am J Roentgenol* 1994;162:437.

# Fundus Calcifications (Optic Disc Drusen and Choroidal Osteoma)

## KEY FACTS

- Fundus calcification represents deposition of calcific hyaline-like material at the surface or deep within the optic disc (often bilateral). Choroidal osteomas are located distal to the optic disc and are more common among patients with tuberous sclerosis.

- Optic disc drusen occur among less than 1% of the population and may be familial.

- When the drusen are deep, they may elevate and blur the margins of the optic disc and clinically mimic papilledema.

- Usually drusen are asymptomatic and incidentally found, but permanent or episodic visual field defects occasionally may be present.

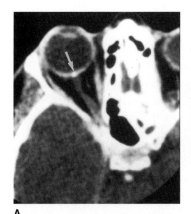
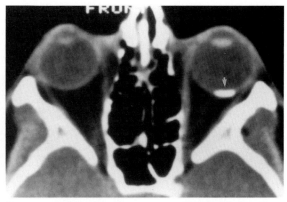

A          B

**FIGURE 30-2**    **(A)** Axial CT scan shows incidentally found focal calcification (*arrow*) in the head of the optic disc. **(B)** Axial CT scan of a different patient shows that the left eye contains a flat calcification (*arrow*) away from the optic nerve head. This is presumed to be a choroidal osteoma.

## Suggested Reading

McNicholas MMJ, Power WJ, Griffin JF. Sonography in optic disk drusen: imaging findings and role in diagnosis when funduscopic findings are normal. *Am J Roentgenol* 1994;162:161.

# *Retinoblastoma (PNET-RB)*

## KEY FACTS

- Retinoblastoma is the most important cause of leukokoria (white pupillary reflex); other causes of leukokoria include persistent hyperplastic primary vitreous, retinopathy of prematurity, congenital cataract, toxocariasis, and Coats' disease.

- The average age at diagnosis is 13 months (most tumors are found before 5 years of age); 40% of cases are hereditary (chromosomal defect in 13q).

- About 25% to 30% of these patients' tumors are bilateral; trilateral retinoblastoma (both eyes and pineal gland or suprasellar region) is very rare.

- If the tumor extends beyond the globe, the mortality rate is near 100%.

- Intraocular calcification is a retinoblastoma until proved otherwise.

- Most patients need enucleation or chemoradiation therapy or both, but newer treatment modalities for small tumors include laser ablation and cryotherapy.

- The overall long-term survival rate is 80%.

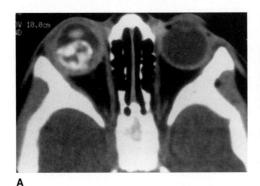 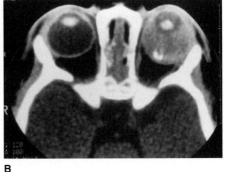

A                                                                B

**FIGURE 30-3**     **(A)** Axial CT scan shows large calcified retinoblastoma in right eye. The posterior sclera is thick, implying invasion by tumor. **(B)** Axial noncontrast CT scan of a different patient shows hyperdense retinoblastoma filling most of the vitreous chamber with a small focus of calcification. The eye is enlarged. In both cases there is no tumor extension outside of the globe.

## Suggested Reading

Hopper KD, Sherman JL, Boal DK, Eggli KD. CT and MR imaging of the pediatric orbit. *Radiographics* 1992;12:485.

# *Orbital Hemangioma (Capillary and Cavernous)*

KEY FACTS

- Capillary hemangioma occurs among children younger than 1 year. It generally is located in the superior nasal quadrant and is an infiltrating lesion that decreases in size with age.

- Cavernous hemangioma is the most common intraconal vascular tumor among adults (mainly in the second to fourth decades of life). It has fibrous pseudocapsule, receives very little blood supply, and may rarely calcify. It can be resected relatively easily.

- Differential diagnosis includes meningioma, schwannoma, and lymphangioma (which are composed of blood vessels, lymphatic channels, occur among young persons and adults and tend to bleed spontaneously).

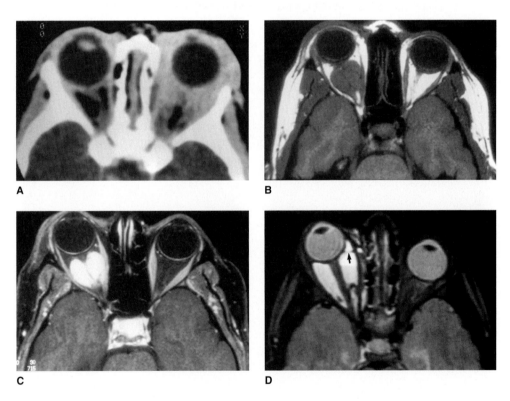

FIGURE 30-4    (A) Axial postcontrast CT scan shows enhancing capillary hemangioma surrounding the left globe and involving both intra- and extraconal compartments. (B) Precontrast axial T1-weighted MR image shows focal intraconal mass surrounding the right optic nerve. There is mild proptosis. This condition did not alter the patient's visual acuity. (C) Corresponding postcontrast fat suppressed T1-weighted image shows that the cavernous hemangioma becomes intensely enhanced. (D) Axial T2-weighted MR image of a different patient shows fluid level (*arrow*) and evidence of old blood products in a right retroocular lymphangioma, which results in proptosis.

## Suggested Reading
Bilaniuk LT, Rapoport RJ. Magnetic resonance imaging of the orbit. *Top Magn Reson Imaging* 1994;6:167.

# *Melanoma*

**KEY FACTS**

- Melanoma arises from the choroid, occurs almost exclusively among white persons, and is the most primary common ocular tumor among adults. It is rare among African Americans.

- Most instances of melanoma are diagnosed clinically and with an ultrasound examination.

- At funduscopic examination melanoma may be difficult to visualize if it is associated with choroid or retinal detachment (especially hemorrhagic detachment).

- Melanoma is most commonly located in the choroid (85%), ciliary body, and iris.

- At CT, melanoma is hyperdense and shows moderate contrast enhancement.

- At MRI, melanoma is classically bright on T1-weighted images and dark on T2-weighted images, and it enhances after contrast administration. Effusions are also well visualized and are slightly bright on T1-weighted MR images, because of the presence of protein and blood, and bright on T2-weighted MR images.

- Differential diagnosis includes choroidal metastases, choroidal hematoma, choroidal or retinal effusion, and inflammatory uveitis.

- The mortality rate reaches 70% when tumor diameter exceeds 12 mm.

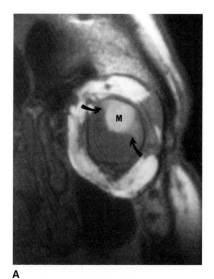

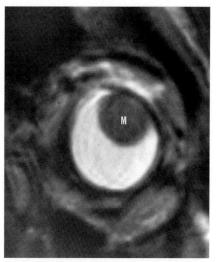

**A**

**B**

## FIGURE 30-5

**(A)** Coronal (surface coil) noncontrast
MR T1-weighted image shows bright
melanoma (*M*) with retinal effusions
(*arrows*). **(B)** Coronal T2-weighted MR
image of the same patient shows the tumor
(*M*) to be dark and effusions to blend with
bright vitreous. **(C)** Axial postcontrast
T1-weighted MR image with fat suppression
shows enhancing melanoma (*arrow*).
(Courtesy of R. M. Quencer, M.D.,
Miami, FL)

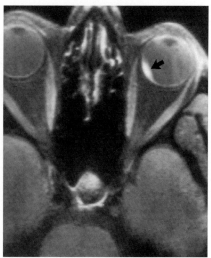

**C**

## Suggested Reading

Mafee MF, Peyman GA, Grisolano JE, et al. Malignant uveal melanoma and simulating
lesions: MR imaging evaluation. *Radiology* 1986;160:773.

# *Lacrimal Gland Masses*

### KEY FACTS

• Enlargement of the lacrimal gland is nonspecific and most often related to viral infection or Sjögren's syndrome (lymphocytic infiltration of tear gland with decreased lacrimation associated with rheumatoid arthritis, lupus, or scleroderma), Mikulicz's syndrome (nonspecific enlargement of salivary and lacrimal glands), sarcoidosis, lymphoma, or leukemia.

• The most common lacrimal gland tumors include benign mixed or pleomorphic tumor (25%), adenoid cystic carcinoma (25%), and lymphoma. Metastasis are rare.

• Dermoids are the most common congenital lesions. Imaging reveals them to be well-defined cyst-like (containing fluid or fat) masses that may be partially calcified and scallop adjacent bones. They are found most often in the region of the frontozygomatic suture in the superolateral aspect of the orbit.

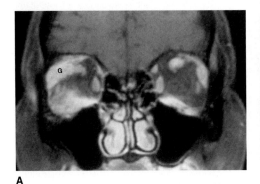
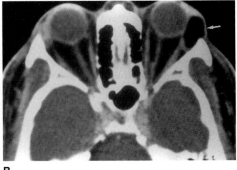

A                                            B

FIGURE 30-6    (A) Coronal postcontrast fat suppressed T1-weighted MR image shows enlarged and enhancing right lacrimal gland (*G*) secondary to sarcoidosis. (B) Axial CT scan shows low-density dermoid (*arrow*) in the left superolateral orbital region.

### Suggested Reading

Warner MA, Weber AL, Jakobiec FA. Benign and malignant tumors of the orbital cavity including the lacrimal gland. *Neuroimaging Clin North Am* 1996;6:123.

# Optic Neuritis

### KEY FACTS

- Optic neuritis is acute inflammation that is usually idiopathic or viral, although it is commonly associated with multiple sclerosis (initial manifestation of multiple sclerosis among 15% of patients). When optic neuritis is caused by multiple sclerosis, 50% of patients show cerebral lesions at MRI.

- Optic neuritis also may be secondary to infections or inflammatory processes of the sinonasal cavities, meninges, and orbital tissues (especially pseudotumor) or to radiation therapy.

- Imaging studies show an enlarged and enhancing nerve. At CT, it may be difficult to differentiate optic neuritis from early perioptic meningioma. MRI of the brain may show periventricular lesions, suggesting multiple sclerosis.

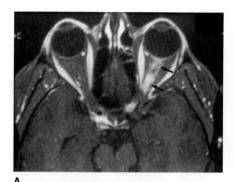 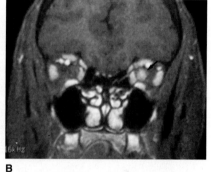

A                                              B

**FIGURE 30-7**     **(A)** Axial postcontrast fat suppressed T1-weighted MR image shows swollen and enhancing left optic nerve (*arrows*) secondary to multiple sclerosis. **(B)** Coronal postcontrast T1-weighted MR image of the same patient shows enhancement of the left optic nerve (*arrow*).

## Suggested Reading

Brodsky MC, Beck RW. The changing role of MR imaging in the evaluation of acute optic neuritis. *Radiology* 1994;192:22.

# *Orbital Pseudotumor*

### KEY FACTS

- Orbital pseudotumor is idiopathic inflammation (although probably related to lymphoma) that affects patients of any age or sex. It presents with painful proptosis.

- The lesion is unilateral in 75% of instances.

- The most common locations are the retroorbital fat, extraocular muscles, optic nerve, sclera, and lacrimal gland.

- Orbital pseudotumor may present as a mass (tumefactive type) or as an enlargement of extraocular muscles (myositic type, which involves the entire muscle including its tendinous attachments).

- It responds readily to steroid therapy.

- It may be associated with Wegener's granulomatosis, fibrosing mediastinitis, autoimmune thyroiditis, and sclerosing cholangitis.

- On T2-weighted MR images, orbital pseudotumor is isointense (remember that malignant growths tend to be hyperintense) and enhances, but lymphoma may appear similar to pseudotumor.

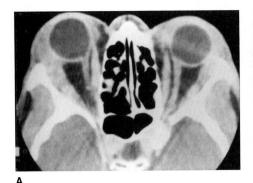 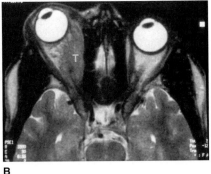

A    B

**F I G U R E   3 0 - 8**    **(A)** Axial CT scan shows that both lateral recti muscles are thick (including their insertions), compatible with the myositic type of pseudotumor. There is bilateral proptosis. **(B)** Axial T2-weighted MR image of a different patient shows tumefactive type of pseudotumor (*T*) involving the right medial rectus muscle and extending into the retroocular fat. The lesion is of low signal intensity.

### Suggested Reading
Weber AL, Jakobiec FA, Sabates NR. Pseudotumor of the orbit. *Neuroimaging Clin North Am* 1996;6:73.

# Graves' Ophthalmopathy

### KEY FACTS

- Graves' ophthalmopathy eventually develops among most patients with Graves' disease but may occur among patients with normal thyroid function. The condition resolves spontaneously in more than 90% of instances (the other patients have eye complications).

- The histologic features of Graves' ophthalmopathy are inflammatory lymphocytic infiltration with edema and deposition of mucopolysaccharides, the end result of which are fibrosis, lipomatosis, and fatty degeneration.

- This condition may lead to optic neuropathy (caused by compression of the optic nerve), diplopia (caused by muscle entrapment), corneal ulcers (caused by proptosis), and conjunctival congestion.

- It may involve any extraocular muscle but most often affects the medial and inferior recti; these muscles may be of high signal intensity on T2-weighted MR images, reflecting edema (the normal diameter of the belly of the recti muscles is 3 mm).

- Graves' ophthalmopathy is the most common cause of proptosis among adults.

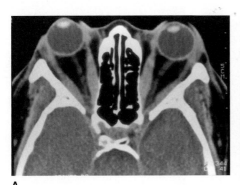 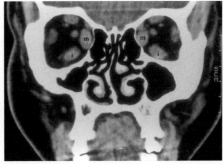

**A**    **B**

**FIGURE 30-9**    **(A)** Axial CT scan shows enlargement of the recti muscles, particularly the medial ones. The insertions are spared. There is bilateral proptosis. **(B)** Coronal CT scan of the same patient shows that all extraocular muscles are large, particularly the medial (*m*) and inferior (*i*) groups.

### Suggested Reading

Weber AL, Dallow RL, Sabates NR. Graves' disease of the orbit. *Neuroimaging Clin North Am* 1996;6:61.

# Orbital Cellulitis and Abscess

### KEY FACTS

- Preseptal cellulitis is a pyogenic inflammation confined to the superficial orbital soft tissues, which are limited posteriorly by the orbital septum (reflection of the periosteum and check ligaments of the eyelids). Treatment usually is medical.

- Postseptal cellulitis is located posterior to the orbital septum. It is usually extraconal and results in subperiosteal phlegmon or abscess. Subperiosteal abscesses are usually secondary to sinonasal (ethmoid) infection, the presence of foreign bodies, and/or fractures. Treatment involves aggressive antibiotic therapy and/or surgical intervention).

- Ophthalmic vein and cavernous sinus septic thrombosis, epidural and subdural empyema, cerebritis, and meningitis are important complications of postseptal inflammation.

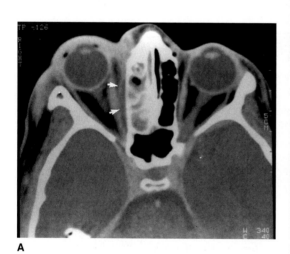
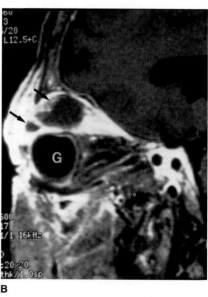

A                                    B

**FIGURE 30-10**    (A) Axial postcontrast CT scan of a child with a right ethmoid sinusitis shows a subperiosteal abscess (*arrows*). There is lateral displacement of the right medial rectus muscle and slight proptosis. (B) Parasagittal postcontrast fat-suppressed T1-weighted MR image of a different patient shows superior orbital multiloculated abscess (*arrows*) secondary to frontal sinusitis. The abscess is extraconal and displaces the globe (*G*) inferiorly.

### Suggested Reading

Towbin R, Han BK, Kaufan RA, Burke M. Postseptal cellulitis: CT in diagnosis and management. *Radiology* 1986;158:735.

# *Detachments and Effusions*

### KEY FACTS

Choroidal:

- Choroidal effusion is accumulation of fluid or blood (postsurgical, trauma, or inflammation) in the subchoroidal space.

- Most choroidal detachments occur in the presence of ocular hypotonia and are caused by increased permeability of choroidal capillaries.

- At imaging, choroidal detachment may be a lenticular or mound-like abnormality.

- Serous effusions are of low signal intensity on T1-weighted MR images and of high signal intensity on T2-weighted MR images. Hemorrhagic and inflammatory effusions may be bright on both T1-weighted and T2-weighted MR images.

Retinal:

- Retinal effusion is accumulation of fluid between the sensory retina and retinal pigment epithelium.

- Rhegmatogenous detachment is caused by a tear in the retina.

- The sensory retina belongs to the central nervous system and therefore does not heal.

- Retinal detachment may result from pulling of the retina (especially among children with retinopathy of prematurity or inflammatory disorders), subretinal hemorrhage caused by trauma, or choroidal lesions.

- At imaging, retinal detachment is commonly V shaped with a small indentation at the level of the optic disc, but it may have any shape, size, or density according to age, cause, and internal organization.

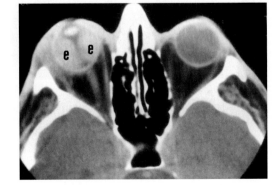

**FIGURE 30-11**
Axial CT scan shows choroidal effusions (*e*), possibly hemorrhagic because of their high density. Note that the effusions stop before the optic nerve head and have a biconvex shape rather the V shape expected with retinal detachment.

### Suggested Reading
Mafee MF, Linder B, Peyman GA, Langer BG, Choi KH, Capek V. Choroidal hematoma and effusion: evaluation with MR imaging. *Radiology* 1988;168:781.

## Ocular Trauma

### KEY FACTS

- Ocular trauma may introduce foreign bodies, or result in hemorrhagic choroidal, or retinal effusion and detachment, dislocation of the lens, hypotonia and collapse from perforations or globe explosions, optic nerve avulsion, hematoma, and extraocular muscle hematoma or entrapment.
- Thin-section CT accurately localizes metallic and nonmetallic foreign bodies.
- At CT, dry wood is hypodense, fresh wood has intermediate to slightly increased density (similar to fresh blood), plastic may be hypo- or hyperdense, and glass is hyperdense.

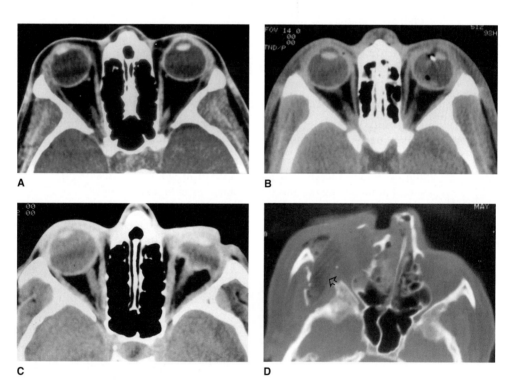

**FIGURE 30-12**    **(A)** Axial CT scan shows collapse of the right anterior chamber (compare with left chamber) indicating perforation and loss of tension in this compartment. **(B)** Axial CT scan shows a left intraocular metallic foreign body, blood and air in the vitreous chamber, and a slight diminution in the size of the globe. **(C)** Axial CT scan shows flat-tire appearance of posterior aspect of left globe secondary to perforation and loss of intraocular tension. **(D)** Axial CT scan (bone window setting) of a patient with multiple facial injuries shows wood fragment (*arrow*) (Courtesy D. Williams, M.D., Winston-Salem, NC).

### Suggested Reading
Asbury CC, Castillo M, Mukherji SK. Review of computed tomographic imaging in acute orbital trauma. *Emerg Radiol* 1995;2:367.

# Index

—Page references for figures are followed by an *f* and page references for tables are followed by a *t*—